# EDITORS' FOREWORD

In most professions there is a traditional gulf between theory and its practice, and nursing is no exception. The gulf is perpetuated when theory is taught in a theoretical setting and practice is taught by the practitioner.

This inherent gulf has to be bridged by students of nursing and publication of this series is an attempt to aid such bridge building.

It aims to help relate theory and practice in a meaningful way whilst underlining the importance of the person being cared for.

It aims to introduce students of nursing to some of the more common problems found in each new area of experience in which they will be asked to work.

It aims to de-mystify some of the technical language they will hear, putting it into context, giving it meaning and enabling understanding.

# ACKNOWLEDGEMENTS

We would like to thank the many people who contributed to the production of this book – the members of the NATN Staffing and Training Committee for their ideas, the nurses who contributed outline care plans and the surgeons who read the care plans.

Not least, thanks are due to Beryl Goodwin and Carol Bracken who had the difficult task of deciphering the writing and fitting all the bits together when typing the manuscript.

The diagram on p. 95 from *The Elements of Nursing* 2nd Edition, by Roper *et al* 1985 is reproduced by kind permission of Churchill Livingstone, Edinburgh.

# CONTENTS

# Introduction

This book, as part of the *Learning to Care* series, considers nursing in the operating department from a different viewpoint than most books about theatre nursing. This change in approach means that some things disappear from view and others come into focus. There are many books about theatre nursing which will tell you about techniques and procedures, such as scrubbing up, checking swabs and laying up trolleys. *Learning to Care in the Theatre* concentrates on the continuing care of the patient whilst in the operating department – on the unique function of the nurse rather than the role of assistant to the surgeon.

# Glossary

Anastomosis
: A connection between two hollow organs, usually to re-establish continuity after removal of a section of, for example, gastro-intestinal tract. Can also be abnormal in a pathological condition.

Disinfection
: Destruction of all *active* micro-organisms, usually by use of heat above 60°C or chemical means.

Endoscope
: A generic term to cover all instruments used to view cavities of internal organs.

Fibre optics
: The use of continuous glass fibres to carry cold light from a remote light source and reflect back images along a separate set of fibres.

Hypoxia
: Reduction in circulating oxygen.

Inhalation anaesthesia
: Anaesthesia administered by the delivery of gases (e.g. nitrous oxide) and volatile liquids (e.g. halothane) with at least 30% oxygen.

Intubation
: Insertion of an endotracheal tube.

Laparotomy
: Incision into the peritoneal cavity.

Muscle relaxant
: Drug used to block the neuromuscular junctions. Produces general paralysis so the patient requires ventilation.

Rectus muscle
: 1  The rectus muscles of the abdomen are two bands of muscle vertically across the abdomen.
  2  The rectus muscles of the eye are the superior, inferior and lateral muscles which move the eye.

Regurgitation
: A silent, passive welling up of stomach contents when the patient is relaxed. Much more dangerous than vomiting which is active.

| Skin antisepsis | It is not possible to sterilise skin, but steps are taken to reduce the microbial flora of the skin by the use of skin preparations, lotions and drapes. |
| --- | --- |
| Sterilisation | Destruction of *all* micro-organisms including *spores*, by the use of pressurised steam (autoclave), irradiation or chemicals. |
| Strangury | Extremely painful retention and difficulty in passing urine. |
| Stridor | The harsh whistling sound of obstructed breathing. NB: Total obstruction is silent. |
| Suture | A stitch. The materials used for sutures and ligatures are the same. |

## Common theatre nomenclature

| Incision | Cutting into. |
| --- | --- |
| Excision | Cutting out – for removal. |
| Resection | Removal of a part of an organ, (e.g. resection of colon). |
| Circumcision | Cutting right around (as for release of the foreskin for phimosis). |
| Retraction | Drawing back the wound edges to give good exposure of the operative site. May be done manually by the assistant using a hand over a pack or hand-held retractor or by the use of a self-retaining retractor. |

## Prefixes

| Adeno- | of glandular tissue. |
| --- | --- |
| Angio- | of vessels, usually but not always, blood vessels. |
| Arthro- | of a joint. |
| Cholecysto- | of the gallbladder. |
| Chondro- | of cartilage. |

| | |
|---|---|
| Colo- | of the colon. |
| Cysto- | of the urinary bladder. |
| Ecto- | outside. |
| Endo- | inside. |
| Pyelo- | of the pelvis or the kidney. |
| Pyloro- | of the pylorus. |
| Pyo- | containing pus. |
| Osteo- | of bone. |
| Retro- | behind. |
| Supra- | above. |

## Suffixes

| | |
|---|---|
| -ectomy | removal of. |
| -gram (graphy) | picture of – usually X-ray picture. |
| -orrhaphy | repair of. |
| -ostomy | opening into – usually permanent or semi-permanent and onto the surface of the skin. |
| -otomy | opening into, during surgery only. |
| -paxy | crushing of – as in lithopaxy |
| -pexy | fixation of – as in orchidopexy. |

(These lists do not include the more common terms with which nurses would be familiar.)

# Welcome to the operating theatre!

Hello, welcome to the operating department, nurse! Like most nurses you are probably feeling a bit scared about your theatre allocation.

The theatre will probably feel very strange to you – only a few nurses take to theatre nursing like a duck to water from the very beginning. You have probably heard lots of horror stories from nurses who have already been to theatre. Don't worry, not only the media exaggerate. American nurses who work in the operating *room* make jokes about working in the 'theatre' in the UK so perhaps we can forgive a few dramatics.

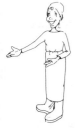

I am sure you already have a lot of questions to ask. Well, we will try to answer them – in fact, we have a few answers for questions you haven't even thought of, as we are quite used to having nurses arrive in theatres who know nothing at all about what happens here.

As a learner you will have worked in many wards where the work follows a similar pattern. In some specialist departments, like Accident & Emergency, Intensive Care or Theatres, life is very different. In the operating department, for instance, all grades of medical, nursing and other staff work together to care for ONE patient at a time.

You may feel unable to relate your previous experience to what you are asked to do in these different departments. Basic common sense and good nursing practice will serve you wherever you are. The working environment in 'theatre' is so different and you may be working more closely with senior medical and nursing staff than you have done before. This may make you a little nervous but you will soon get used to working as part of the theatre team in more informal relationships.

The theatre team is a real team, not just a group of people working together. Notice how each person is doing something different but how each of his or her duties interlocks and is dependent on what other team members are doing. Timing and good working relationships are vital to the efficient working of a team.

## Why are you coming to the operating department?

Some countries do not include the operating department experience in nursing training. You may yourself be wondering why you are required to come to the operating department during your training. Perhaps we should consider the aims for this allocation.

1  The surgical patient's experience does not stop at the ward door. It includes what happens in the operating department. Spending some time there gives you deeper insight into the reasons for carrying out pre-operative care meticulously, according to your ward procedures. It will also help you understand any problems that the patient may have post-operatively.
2  Developing good communications between the ward and the operating department for patient safety and good nursing care. You may never work there again but you will have an understanding of the theatre nurses' problems and priorities.
3  You will receive training and experience in the care of the unconscious and highly dependent patient.
4  The maintenance of infection control and asepsis is vital in the operating theatre.

Experience of theatre aseptic technique will always be of use to you in your future career as a nurse.
5 You will also gain insight into the maintenance of safety for both staff and patients.
6 There are opportunities to learn about the maintenance of homeostasis including fluid replacement, pain control and the control of patient anxiety.


## Aim of the theatre experience

In order to participate with understanding in the total care of the surgical patient, you will be helped and guided to acquire and develop the skills, knowledge and attitudes necessary to meet the needs of patients in the pre-operative, intra-operative and immediate post-operative period.

**Objectives (National Association of Theatre Nurses 1982)**
At the end of the experience, the learner will be able to:–
1 List the necessary observations required to assess a patient's condition prior to procedures under anaesthesia.
2 Safely care for the patient before, during and after anaesthesia.
3 Participate effectively as a member of a multi-disciplinary team responsible for the patient's nursing care and management while in the operating department.
4 Carry out all precautions to safeguard patients and staff.
5 Use the appropriate skills to facilitate effective communication.
6 Administer appropriate nursing care to the patient during the immediate post-operative period.
7 Discuss the underlying principles of good operating department design, organisation and management.

At the beginning of this experience it is essential to become familiar with:–
1 The layout of the theatre area and the health and safety measures provided.
2 The theatre routine and organisation, particularly

with regard to theatre dress, changing facilities and
duty schedules.
3   Positioning of fire points and fire escape routes.
4   The location of emergency equipment.
5   The procedure to be followed in emergency
situations.
6   Legal implications for patients and staff relevant to
the theatre area.
7   Special circumstances associated with the clinical
area.

## The nursing process in the operating theatre

When you first arrive in the department it may
seem a very technical environment where
little nursing care is carried out. However this
is not so, for there is great scope for nursing
care of patients within the operating department.

You will already be familiar with the concept of the Nursing Process from your ward
experience. The same concept provides an
ideal way of approaching the care of a patient
in the operating theatre during a time when
patients are probably at their most vulnerable.

In order to provide nursing care suitable to
meet individual patients' needs, the theatre
nurse requires information about the patient.
Some of the information is already available so
good communication between ward staff and
theatre staff is essential. The ward nurse can
convey the special needs of each patient to the
theatre nurse. For example, the emaciated
patient who will require special preparation of
the operating table to reduce the risk of pressure sore development during the operation, or
the patient with rheumatoid arthritis for
whom table adaptation may be necessary to
achieve the required position for surgery because of stiff joints.

Alternatively, the theatre nurse may collect

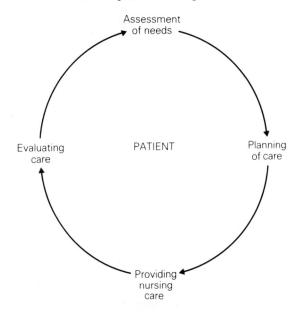

the required information needed to plan care by carrying out a *pre-operative visit.* This involves the theatre nurse visiting the patient on the ward during the pre-operative period in order to assess the patient's needs. It also allows the patient to ask the theatre nurse questions about his visit to theatre which the ward nurses may not be able to answer.

The visit also enables the patient to identify with a member of the theatre staff so that on the day of operation, there is one familiar face to greet him. Ideally, the theatre nurse who carries out the pre-operative visit should be the nurse who receives the patient into theatre. A familiar face reduces anxiety levels for the patient and provides an added safety factor when the patient is checked in to theatre as the nurse is able to identify the patient.

The visiting theatre nurse can give the patients accurate information about what to expect when they arrive in the reception area and the anaesthetic room and when they wake up in the recovery room following their operation. Patients may ask about post-operative pain and the availability of analgesia to control it; whether they will have an intravenous infusion; the position of the wound or the type of dressing and if there will be any drainage. Research has shown that the well-informed patient has a smoother, uncomplicated post-operative recovery following surgery, in comparison to the patient who has minimal knowledge of what is to happen before, during and following surgery (Boore 1978).

By using the concept we call the Nursing Process, continuity of care can be achieved as the patient progresses from the operating room to the recovery room. There is a written nursing record of the care which has been given to meet the patient's individual needs as he moves from one area of the operating department to the next and from one group of nursing staff to another.

Post-operative recovery needs can be planned for individual patients and the patient's recovery recorded. This will include information about pain assessment and any analgesia given as well as recordings of assessment of cardiovascular and respiratory functions made by the recovery room nurse. Drainage from wound drains and fluid replacement recordings will also be made as applicable.

An initial evaluation of the care given to the patient in theatre can be done in the recovery room; for example, the inspection of pressure points for signs of redness.

To carry out a full evaluation of patient care in theatre, it is probably better if the theatre nurse pays a post-operative visit to the ward when the patient has recovered sufficiently to participate fully in the evaluation.

THE NURSING PROCESS IN THE OPERATING DEPARTMENT

1 **Pre-operative visit** by theatre nurse to collect data.
2 **Assessment** of patient's needs during operation.
3 **Planning** of care by theatre nurse in readiness to receive the patient in theatre.
4 **Providing nursing care** in reception area
   – anaesthetic room
   – operating room
   – recovery room.
5 **Evaluating** care and handing patient over to ward nurse.
6 **Longer term evaluation** carried out during *post-operative ward visit*.

It should be noted that not all theatres use a nursing process approach to nursing care in the operating theatre. You, as a student or pupil nurse will, however, be receiving your nurse training using a problem solving approach – and probably your training is based on a nursing model.

A nursing model is, of course, a conceptual model and as such, contains a representation of everything involved in nursing and how these elements relate. Each model approaches these elements in a different way and one model is more appropriate in, say, the community or long-stay ward whilst another model will be more appropriate for the theatre or intensive therapy unit (ITU). We have more to say about models in Chapter 7 – Writing a Care Study.

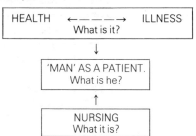

In many theatres you will be able to 'follow' one patient right through his theatre experience – from ward to ward as it were – and will probably follow this by writing up a care study.

Even if your theatres are not implementing an individualised approach to the planning of care, there may be a standard pre-operative check list. *Do not confuse this with an assessment or care plan.* It is purely what it says it is, a check list to allow ward nurses to inform theatre nurses what they have done and is more related to the safety of the patient than to individualised patient care.

# 2 Starting to work in theatre

To help you know a little more about how operating theatres actually function, we will start with the general daily routine. When you come on duty you will report to the senior nurse or the nurse specifically designated to look after you. At this stage you may be one of a group of nurses who are all starting their theatre allocation together or there may be just you in your particular theatre. The nurse looking after you will explain which theatre, anaesthetic room or recovery area you are to work in. These are the three areas in which you are to gain experience. She will take you to your working area and introduce you to the people with whom you will be working.

## Entering the operating theatre

The staff changing room is the place where you will change from your ordinary clothes into theatre dress. The nurse looking after you, usually a sister, will take you into the changing room where you will be issued with shoes and allocated a locker in which to place your things. Always lock away any money or valuables. You will be shown how to wear your cap and mask, dress or trouser suit and shoes.

At this time you will also be reminded of the need for scrupulous personal hygiene including special attention to hair and nails and attention to bathing and underwear changes. Inadequate personal hygiene may be very oppressive when in close proximity for several hours – and so can heavy perfume or after-shave.

Theatre uniform may be colour coded to identify different grades of staff or colour coded hats may be used. When surgeons and anaesthetists come and go in different theatres, it is important for them to be able to identify a competent person in an emergency. You, and anybody else new to the theatre may, for example, wear a white cap so that no-one will expect you to know what you cannot know yet.

When you change into your theatre clothes, you first of all remove your outer clothes, cover your hair with a theatre hat, then put on your dress or trouser suit. Putting your hat on first prevents bacterial contamination of your clean theatre clothes. Your shoes will be special anti-static shoes. It is important for them to fit comfortably – you could be standing still for a long time – and you will be on your feet for even longer.

**REMEMBER**
**Wearing theatre clothes correctly is one of the important steps in setting a high standard of infection control in the operating theatre.**
Before entering the theatre suite CHECK that:–
1  Your hair is completely covered.
2  You are wearing theatre dress correctly.
3  You have removed all your jewellery.
4  Your shoes are comfortable.
5  You have locked away anything of value.
6  You have got your key safely!

It is not necessary to wear a mask until you enter the operating theatre itself. The mask itself should feel comfortable and, once in place, should not be fingered. To function properly it must be worn properly.

**Donning a mask**
1  Remove mask from box – handle by tapes as far as possible.
2  If the type with plastic band at one side, fit this band over the nose comfortably.

3   Tie the top tapes on top of the head.
4   Tie the bottom tapes round your neck.
5   The mask should fit closely.
6   Do not touch or 'wiggle' your mask.

**Removing a mask**
1   Remove *by tapes* and drop straight into rubbish bin.
2   Do not crumple mask in hand.
3   Do not put mask in pocket.
4   Do not allow mask to hang under chin.

## Inside the theatre suite

You are now ready to enter the CLEAN AREA –
you may only go into the clean areas of a
theatre when wearing correct theatre dress.
Sister's office is probably in the clean area so
this is when your guide and mentor may show
you the rotas and request books and explain
the policy for reporting staff sickness.

A tour of the department will now follow.
Explanations in each area will be brief and
simple as too much detail at this stage will just
confuse you. You will also see the rest rooms
and be told what refreshments are available
and the times for coffee and meal breaks.

## The theatre staff

When you arrive in your allocated area there
are bound to be different grades of staff for you
to get to know. There are many people working in an operating department but they are all
necessary for the care of the patients who are,
after all, the most important people in
theatres. The staff are allocated to give the
correct 'mix' of experience and skills. There is
also a very high percentage of nurses – sisters,
staff nurses and enrolled nurses, all apparently
very skilled and confident. As well as caring
for the patient they are also there to give you

help and guidance in learning their special skills. Don't worry about working so much more closely with senior nurses, surgeons and anaesthetists. You will soon see that no-one

The theatre staff. The anaesthetist could also be included.

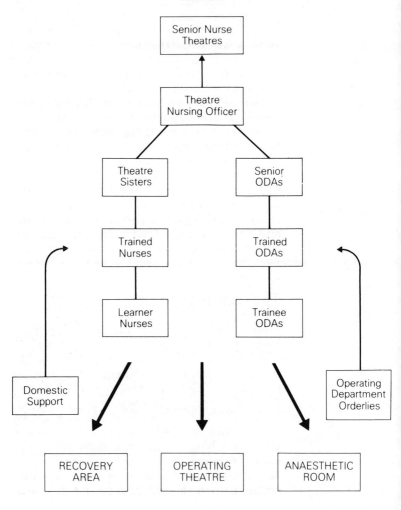

can work in isolation here and that good surgery needs good team work.

*Please do ask questions*
If you show interest and ask questions, most doctors are more than happy to explain what they are doing and why, but choose your moment with care. It is wise to remember that patients may still be able to hear and remember a conversation even if they are apparently unconscious. Also bear in mind that the surgeon and anaesthetist carry total responsibility for the patient during surgery and anaesthesia and will not appreciate being interrupted at a crucial moment.

You will also work with the Operating Department Assistants (ODAs). Most of them are men but more girls are beginning to enjoy this work as well. ODAs have a two-year training in all the practical theatre skills which theatre nurses have. In some hospitals they have a major role in assisting the anaesthetist, although not in all.

Also working as permanent staff in the theatres are Operating Department Orderlies (ODOs). These are the theatre porters who are responsible for transporting and lifting patients.

Some theatres have Theatre Sterile Supply Unit (TSSU) staff stationed in the theatre as well as in the Central Sterile Supply Department (CSSD) itself – and we must not forget the domestic staff who keep us fed, clothed and watered.

A tip – people usually write their names on the back of their theatre shoes – so have a quick look to remind yourself who someone is.

# Geography of an operating theatre

The theatre you will be working in may be a single or twin theatre suite or part of a large complex. Whatever their design, all theatres have certain features in common.

**Barriers:** These vary from a line painted on the floor to a solid wall which can only be passed through special doors or through an air lock. DO observe any notices on doors.

**'Clean' and 'Dirty' Areas:** Everyone and everything which comes into theatres must be **clean**. There are **flow patterns** through the theatre. Always **from clean → to dirty → out**.

Once anything is contaminated, or regarded as 'dirty' it must be discarded or recycled. Dirty things go out through a separate 'dirty' exit. Nothing comes back in until it has been recycled by washing and sterilisation. Staff are not often discarded! They are 'recycled' by washing and changing!

**Operating Theatre Layout:** There are a number of different designs for an operating theatre. An example is shown opposite. Each theatre consists of the theatre itself, an anaesthetic room, preparation room, 'scrub up' room and a 'dirty' utility room.

Standard operating room furniture includes the operating table, lights, diathermy machine used by the surgeon to control bleeding points, X-ray viewing box, swab board and swab rack for checking swabs and the anaesthetic machine. There are also a number of stools as for some operations the surgeon needs to sit down. All rubber wheels, covers and shoes are made of special anti-static rubber to prevent the build up of 'static'.

## Ventilation of an operating theatre

All theatres have a separate ventilation system which pumps **clean** filtered air into the cleanest part of the operating theatre. The air

Layout of an operating theatre. In an older theatre without CSSD back-up, there are autoclaves, sluice and more storage space.

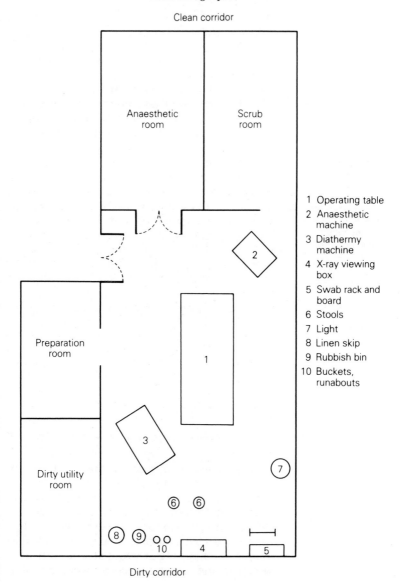

Clean corridor

Anaesthetic room

Scrub room

Preparation room

Dirty utility room

Dirty corridor

1 Operating table
2 Anaesthetic machine
3 Diathermy machine
4 X-ray viewing box
5 Swab rack and board
6 Stools
7 Light
8 Linen skip
9 Rubbish bin
10 Buckets, runabouts

is pumped into the theatre so that the air pressure is higher inside than outside. This means that air always flows out of the theatre preventing dirty air from the rest of the hospital getting in. The most commonly used ventilation system gives an entire change of air 20 times in an hour. In theatres which need to be exceptionally clean, such as some orthopaedic theatres, a special **laminar air flow** system blows streams of air down or across the patient, changing the air up to 300 times in an hour. The engineers and the microbiologists check the cleanliness of the air by doing particle counts. The controls of the ventilation system also control the **humidity** and the **temperature**.

**A particle count** checks particles the size of bacteria. A theatre cannot be used if the particle count is too high. It is always done before opening a new theatre or after repairs.

The air humidity is important to prevent static electricity building up. We cannot afford to have sparks in theatre as we do still occasionally use flammable anaesthetics and we certainly use volatile liquids (alcohol, spirit) regularly. The temperature is controlled to ensure a comfortable environment both for staff and to maintain the patient's temperature. Only if we are operating on newly born babies or very old patients do we need to keep the theatre very warm.

## Communications

When you first work in the operating theatre you will probably experience some difficulty with personal communications, particularly in hearing what people are saying. This is because everyone is wearing a mask and cap which tends to stop you hearing what they are saying, and you are used to seeing peoples' lips moving as they speak. You may feel that people are shouting at you. Have no fear, this will pass and you will become accustomed to

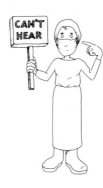

communicating with colleagues irrespective of these drawbacks.

You will find that people in theatre use non-verbal clues particularly when scrubbed. Whilst asking for an item they may point to a similar item they already have, or hold up an item, such as a suture packet, to show the colour code. People also use their eyes to indicate in which direction you need to move to find the item concerned. If you use your eyes too, you will find these non-verbal clues very helpful.

The language in theatres can also be a bit overpowering. By that, it doesn't mean that the air is blue, though it can be, but you may hear many terms and phrases you have not heard before. So – if you are asked to do something you do not understand, say so. Ask questions and be inquisitive and before long you will understand the language more clearly.

During your time in theatre you will be required to take messages and telephone calls. When answering the telephone:

1  State your location – 'Theatre 2 . . .'
2  State your name and grade – 'Student Nurse Anyperson'.

This is helpful to the person at the other end who may have a complicated or important message. When you take a message, write it down. It may appear to be quite short but can turn out to be longer and longer and you will feel foolish if you have to ask them to repeat the whole message.

When giving a message to the surgeon, it is accepted practice to do so through the scrub nurse at an appropriate moment. She is in the best position to ascertain if the surgeon is concentrating particularly hard on a difficult stage of the operation. She will pass on the message or ask the surgeon to speak to you. An anaesthetist can often come to the telephone where a surgeon cannot, as long as there is an anaesthetic assistant available to look after the patient.

## Stress

We have already said that relationships in theatre are fairly relaxed and informal but tempers can flare if something is not going well. Things can go wrong quickly and need quick reactions. Often it is the surgeon who gets edgy – he carries ultimate responsibility for the patient's safety – and he's the one doing the operation. This can affect the whole team though a good theatre nurse defuses the situation by remaining calm and doing the right thing quickly. At times like this, people don't have time to be polite. They just need the right equipment and the right response quickly. Just do what you are asked to do quietly and quickly and keep a low profile – it will all be back to normal over a cup of tea afterwards.

## Fainting

Whilst we are talking about stress, it might be as well to consider the question of fainting. Before you come to the theatre you may hear stories about people fainting at the prospect of seeing operations. The vast majority of operations are not bloody or unpleasant to watch. The reasons for fainting can be standing still for a long time, not having any breakfast, getting too hot or the tension of being in a new place where you don't know what to expect. Exactly the same reasons, in fact, why a guardsman faints on the Queen's birthday parade.

So:

– eat breakfast before coming on duty
– flex your calf muscles if standing still for a
  long time
– tell the staff if you have a tendency to faint.

If you do feel funny – you usually start to feel hot and sick – go out of theatre and sit down. A cup of tea or a glass of water can help. After a little while you will feel better. Of course, there will always be some wag who will tell you 'If you must faint, fall backwards' – that is away from the operation.

## Claustrophobia

Quite a few modern theatres do not have windows. Working in a windowless environment in an unaccustomed cap and mask can feel very confusing and strange but you will get used to it very quickly. Just a few people suffer from real claustrophobia and may need to get out of theatre at intervals until they have acclimatised. Do speak to theatre sister or your tutor if you have problems with claustrophobia. It may be possible to allocate you to a theatre with windows.

# 3 Theatre nursing practice

## The sterile field

When you hear theatre nurses talk about 'the sterile field', they mean the area immediately surrounding the patient once he has been covered with sterile drapes. It includes the scrub nurse's trolleys, and all 'scrubbed' personnel. In short, everything covered by sterile drapes and everyone wearing sterile gowns and gloves. The drapes and gowns are usually green (linen) or blue (disposable). Nobody except the 'scrub team' is allowed within the sterile field without the express instructions of the scrub nurse or surgeon, to avoid accidental contamination. All materials used in the sterile field are sterilised.

The basic team for an operation consists of three medical members and three theatre staff. It can include more for some types of surgery. The surgeon may not have a doctor to assist for emergency surgery during the night so a qualified member of the theatre staff may assist. Within the team, there is also the smaller 'scrubbed' team. This is the surgeon, his assistant and the nurses who have 'scrubbed up', put on sterile gloves and gowns and are using aseptic technique to handle sterilised equipment. The *scrub nurse's* job is to prepare and control the instruments, swabs and other equipment.

Two good phrases to remember are:
*'Be conscious of your margins of safety'*
and
*'Develop a good surgical conscience'*
This means that you should always be aware of the limits

# The theatre team

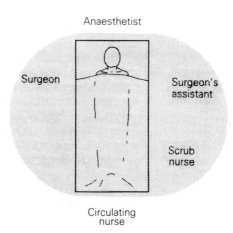

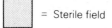 = Sterile field

Anaesthetic
assistant

Anaesthetist

Surgeon

Surgeon's
assistant

Scrub
nurse

Circulating
nurse

of the sterile field, whether scrubbed or not, and you must always know whether something is sterile and SAY so if you contaminate something.

**Aseptic technique**
Technique using sterile materials to prevent contamination of surgical wound by micro-organisms. Also involves antiseptic preparation of patient's skin, and hands of staff.

This way we maintain a good theatre aseptic technique.

## Knowing what to get

There is a vast amount of equipment and stored supplies in an operating suite. You will find that there are a number of guides to finding things:
- Store rooms will be clearly labelled, perhaps with an index or plan available.
- All the equipment which the theatre nurses expect to use during an operating session will be in the theatre.

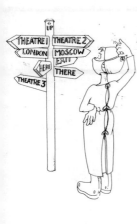

– A record of both surgeons' and anaesthetists' needs (and likes and dislikes) will be kept as a Kardex or in a book.

## Specimens

During the operation the surgeon may remove pieces of tissue for histological or bacteriological examination. It is very important to have the correct container available. You will be shown how to use these and how to label the specimen container – not the lid! – after the specimen is in the container. The laboratory form must be completed and signed by the doctor, before both specimen and form leave the theatre. A register is kept of all specimens.

## Documents

The patient's notes come to the theatre with him and the surgeon will 'write up' the operation in the notes. The main theatre record is the **operations register** which is maintained by the theatre nurses and is used also for statistical purposes. You will be shown how this is filled in and signed by the 'scrub' and circulating nurses. It is essential that the register is correctly completed.

## Confidentiality

The patient is entitled to confidentiality in the operating theatre, just as elsewhere in the hospital, so do be careful that you do not breach that confidentiality when you are discussing interesting operations.

## Drugs

In the recovery area the same rules apply for the storage, use and administration of Controlled Drugs as in other wards. In the anaesthetic room and theatre the anaesthetist administers these drugs so theatre nurses are responsible only for storing and accounting for the stock drugs.

## Disposal of used equipment

You will find that the disposal of linen, sharps and rubbish will be similar to ward procedures, except that **theatre rubbish and linen is always regarded as contaminated**.
- DO observe the colour coding for linen and rubbish bags.
- DO use sharps boxes correctly.
- DO follow the theatre procedure for recycling instruments.
- DO put rubbish into the correct bag or container.
- DO make sure that rubbish bags are tied securely.

## Infected patients

There will be clearly defined procedures for infected patients in your theatre. Most of the patients which we treat as 'infected' are not infectious until the operation starts. There are two groups of infected patients:

1  A patient with an abscess which yields pus when opened. This can contaminate instruments and equipment. In this case we only have to worry about getting the instruments to the Theatre Sterile Supply Unit safely to be autoclaved before anyone

handles them. Theatre Sterile Supply Unit is part of the Central Sterile Supply Department (CSSD).

2 A patient for surgery who has a blood-borne infection which could be dangerous to staff, for example, Hepatitis B. For these virus infections, it is advisable to use disposable drapes and gowns and take precautions to protect other staff from blood contamination. The patient is usually a carrier and not in the active stage of the disease.

This means that we have two slightly different procedures for dealing with infected patients. You will be shown what to do – don't worry, the rest of the theatre team will be there as well. As a learner, you should not be present when 'high risk' infectious patients are undergoing surgery.

> DO NOT HANDLE BLOODSTAINED MATERIAL WITH BARE HANDS — USE FORCEPS OR WEAR GLOVES.

## Safety in the operating department

Safety has always been a byword in the operating department for both patients and staff. You will find that theatre nurses are very conscious of safety codes. You will be asked to read the theatre policy and procedures before you enter the theatre. These include the local Health & Safety policies and the Joint Memoranda. The Joint Memoranda are two books produced jointly by the RCN and Medical Defence Union to outline codes of practice for patient identification and to prevent foreign bodies being left in a patient. You will also be required to know the fire and emergency procedures in your theatre. A number of procedures relating to your personal safety will be drawn to your attention.

### X-rays in theatre

You must follow the theatre procedure to reduce exposure to X-rays to a minimum. This means keeping a safe distance when X-rays are taken, protecting yourself with a wall, a lead screen or lead waistcoat if you cannot leave the immediate vicinity of the X-rays. Pregnant nurses must not be in the theatre when X-rays are being used.

### Anaesthetic gases

As there is a statistically higher incidence of certain conditions amongst theatre nurses and anaesthetists, most theatres now have 'scavenger systems' which directly extract expired anaesthetic gases from the theatre. The most significant condition related to anaesthetic gases was a statistically higher incidence of spontaneous abortions in female nurses and anaesthetists so pregnant nurses are given the opportunity to work elsewhere.

### Pregnancy

Because of these risks you must discuss the matter with the nurse in charge of theatre or your tutor if there is any possibility that you are pregnant.

### Accidents

The accident procedures are the same as the rest of the hospital, but the commonest theatre accident is a cut or prick from a scalpel blade or needle. If you do cut your finger, **report it at once**. If the needle or blade has been used, the patient's name must be recorded on the accident form as a safeguard.

> If you come on duty with a cut on your hand – report it to sister. That applies also to any other possible source of infection such as a sore throat. Sister will make the decision as to whether you are at risk or a possible infection risk to others.

# Communications with other departments

It takes a great deal of organisation to arrange the simultaneous arrival, in a prepared fully-staffed theatre, of the patient, the supplies, the surgeon and the anaesthetist – as well as any other people such as radiographers or laboratory technicians. Some of the planning is done in advance by written duty rotas, allocation of surgeons' sessions and written orders. To allow for last minute changes and emergencies, the telephone is very important. You may become involved in this network when you answer the telephone. Never take a message about theatre bookings or cancellations – always refer it to the sister in charge. She is the only person who has the full picture. It is very embarrassing to tell sister that the houseman has booked an appendix for 6 o'clock and she 'hits the roof' because one list is running late and she has no staff to open another theatre!

**Theatre Sterile Supply Unit (TSSU)**
This is probably the most important back up unit to the smooth running of theatres because no theatre can run without its sterile supplies. It is virtually an extension of the operating theatre, usually close by if not inside the department and managed by a former theatre sister or senior ODA.

**Radiography**
A radiography department usually has at least one radiographer responsible for surgical X-rays carried out during surgery, as well as the surgical X-rays procedure carried out in the department itself. We have to make sure that we book the radiographer for the right time – and inform her of any change – so as not to waste her time. This can also work the other way. If we do not have the radiographer there

Communication routes. This diagram will help you to understand the importance of a good framework of written information and how the nurse in charge of theatre uses verbal communications in response to changes.

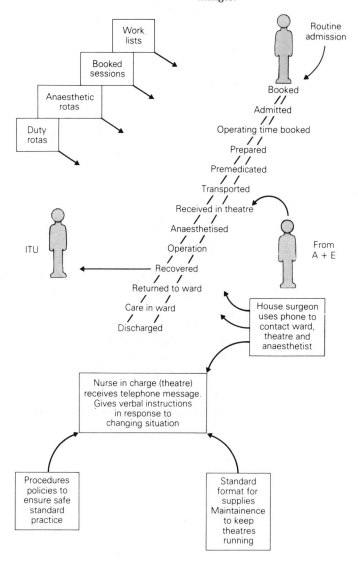

Communications with other departments.

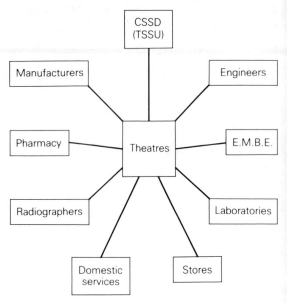

at the right time, we may have to prolong the anaesthetic which is not good for the patient.

**Engineers**
In addition to the hospital engineers and electricians who keep the basic services going, theatres have a lot of work for EBME (electro-bio-medical engineers) who look after the anaesthetic and diathermy machines as well as other equipment. They maintain and repair essential and expensive equipment to keep the theatres running.

# 4 Assessment and planning of the care of the patient during the peri-operative period

Theatre nurses think of the time in which patients are in their care as 'the peri-operative time' so we will use that expression. It means before, during and after surgery.

## Standard care plans

As every patient is coming to the operating department for an operation, there is a very good case for developing standard care plans to avoid constantly re-writing the same details in the nursing notes. When we subject patients to the hazards of surgery there are a number of common problems in each area of the operating department, so we can apply the problem solving approach to the situation as well as to the care of individual patients.

In an ideal situation, a pre-operative visit would ensure that the patient meets and is assessed by the nurse who will receive him into the department and will be available to recover the patient. Failing this, the theatre nurse will assess the patient on arrival in the theatre. She will, of course, receive some information in advance from the operation list and perhaps from the medical staff or ward nurses, but this may not relate to the person but to the surgical problem. We can however draw up a standard care plan for the situation –

for any operation – before we assess the individual patient's needs. This will cover a considerable amount of the nursing care for every patient. But do remember – a pre-operative check list is not a care plan.

Take a look at the three following standard care plans for:

1  nursing care in the anaesthetic room,
2  nursing care during an operation,
3  nursing care during the recovery period.

NB: These are suggested basic care plans which will require extension to meet individual patients' needs.

Now turn to the case studies of individual patients to see how the standard care plans are developed to identify individual needs and the planning of nursing actions. This is a time when the patient is extremely vulnerable and many nursing actions are directed to ensuring patient safety and the protection of his rights as a person.

Each care study concentrates on one aspect of patient care in the operating theatre and does not include all the care included in the standard care plan.

**Nursing Care in the Anaesthetic Room**

| POTENTIAL PROBLEM | OUTCOME | NURSING ACTION | RATIONALE |
|---|---|---|---|
| Ensuring that the correct patient has the right operation. | The patient undergoes the operation to which he has consented. | Methodical check of the patient's identification bracelet and documents. Address the patient by name. | Many patients are passing through the care of several groups of nurses. |
| Anxiety due to inadequate explanation and stress of surgery. | Pre-op anxiety reduced to a level with which the patient can cope without distress. | Establish a rapport with the patient and give appropriate explanations and physical support. Ensure that the patient understands what is said to him. | 1 To make sure the patient can hear and see to receive explanation and verbal support. 2 To ensure that the patient is as able as possible to cope with the physical stress of surgery. |
| Hazards of inducing anaesthesia. | Patient will have a safe and uneventful induction. | Check the essential equipment is clean, available and in working order. Establish time of last intake of food and fluid. Check for loose or capped or solitary teeth. Check premedication was given as prescribed. Be aware of existing medical conditions, allergies or drug regimes. | 1 There is no time to replace or find equipment during induction. 2 The patient's airway is vulnerable during induction. 3 The anaesthetic regime can be complicated by patient reactions. |

**Nursing Care in the Anaesthetic Room** – *contd.*

| POTENTIAL PROBLEM | OUTCOME | NURSING ACTION | RATIONALE |
|---|---|---|---|
| Hazards of undergoing surgery. | Uneventful recovery from surgery. | Check that the pre-op shave has been done. Check that skin/bowel or other preparations have been carried out adequately. Ensure that any special equipment has arrived with the patient. | These checks must be completed *before* the operation commences. |
| Accidental injury whilst sedated or anaesthetised. | Operation completed with no untoward incident or accidental injury. | Ensure stretcher canvas correctly positioned under patient and in good condition. Take care to avoid injury when inserting stretcher poles and lifting. Position the patient to avoid pressure injuries. | The patient is not able to speak for himself or move to relieve discomfort or potentially dangerous pressure on skin, nerves or blood vessels. |

## Nursing Care During an Operation

| POTENTIAL PROBLEM | OUTCOME | NURSING ACTION | RATIONALE |
|---|---|---|---|
| Wound infection | Satisfactory healing of surgical wound by first intention healing. | Prepare and present sterile equipment and material using good theatre aseptic technique. | The patient's defences are breached by surgery and his resistance lowered due to the stress of surgery or his illness. |
| Diathermy or pressure injury. | Operation safely completed without incidental harm to the patient. | Ensure patient correctly and safely supported. Observe the patient throughout the operation to ensure that he remains safe. Use diathermy and other equipment according to manufacturer's instructions and safety rules. | 1 Length of time is important in development of pressure injuries. 2 Patient is covered by drapes and position can change during surgery. 3 Equipment may not be safe unless used correctly. |
| Failure to remove swabs, needles, instruments from the wound. | No foreign bodies retained in wound after closure. | Carry out meticulous swab, needle and instrument counts before, during and after surgery according to established procedures. | A great many swabs, needles and instruments may be used. They may not be visible and could be forgotten if not counted. |

**Nursing Care During an Operation** – *contd.*

| POTENTIAL PROBLEM | OUTCOME | NURSING ACTION | RATIONALE |
|---|---|---|---|
| Inadequate documentation and communication of patient information. | Correct documentation of all care given to the patient in the peri-operative period. | Record all nursing actions and patient responses to treatment. Ensure that theatre register is correctly completed. | To ensure that reference can be made to occurrences in theatre and to ensure good communication between theatre, recovery and the ward. |
| Lack of respect for the person undergoing theatre procedures. | Patient's dignity will be maintained throughout the operation. | Avoid excessive exposure. Avoid depersonalisation of the patient. Take care in choice of words in conversations around the unconscious patient. | It is important to maintain the patient's right to respect as a person throughout the operations of surgery and anaesthesia. |

## Nursing Care of the Patient During the Recovery Period

| POTENTIAL PROBLEM | OUTCOME | NURSING ACTION | RATIONALE |
|---|---|---|---|
| Airway obstruction. | Uncomplicated return to independent respiration. | Maintain patency of airway by positioning and/or jaw support until cough and swallowing reflexes return. Check that suction equipment is working and oxygen available. | Patient cannot guard his own airway until his swallowing and cough reflexes return. This is a time when good oxygenation is essential. |
| Fluid loss or bleeding. | Early recognition of changes in vital signs to prevent or reverse symptoms of hypovolaemic shock. | Carry out regular observations and monitoring of vital signs. Record and report as necessary<br>– Colour<br>– Respiration<br>– Pulse<br>– Blood pressure<br>– Temperature<br>– Fluid intake<br>– Fluid output<br>– Wound and other drainage.<br>Specific postoperative checks.<br>Peripheral temperatures.<br>General warmth. | 1 Continuous monitoring and observation will ensure early recognition of changes in the patient's general condition following surgery.<br>2 Specific checks will be ordered for any 'high risk' hazards. |
| Postoperative pain. | Reduction of pain to a minimum. | Monitor pain levels by observation of restlessness and verbal reports from the patient.<br>Give analgesia as prescribed.<br>Monitor and record effects and effectiveness of pain relief. | Maintaining the patient pain free reduces anxiety and physical stress. |

39

**Nursing Care of the Patient During the Recovery Period** – *contd.*

| POTENTIAL PROBLEM | OUTCOME | NURSING ACTION | RATIONALE |
|---|---|---|---|
| Accidental injury whilst recovering from anaesthesia/analgesia. | Uneventful recovery without accidental injury or incident. | Ensure safety rails in position. Constant nursing vigilance. Check patient's position to ensure comfort and safety. Assessment of conscious state. | The patient is in an unstable and vulnerable state until he regains full consciousness. |
| Postoperative anxiety and over-stimulation. | Smooth and natural recovery from anaesthesia. | Reassure the patient that the operation is over. Keep the patient quiet and avoid unnecessary disturbance. Explain nursing actions. Be aware that hearing returns before other signs of returning consciousness. | The patient may be more aware than he appears or may recover rather slowly, tempting the nurse to stimulate him into showing signs of consciousness. |
| Lack of continuity of care. | Safe return to the ward and continuance of good post opcare. | Complete documentation of all care given during peri-operative period. Record patient responses. | Verbal reports at handover can be misinterpreted or forgotten. |

# 5 Mrs Stonehouse has a cholecystectomy

## HISTORY

**The gallbaldder** stores and concentrates bile produced in the liver. Bile is released in response to cholecystokinin and duodenal peristalsis. It aids digestion and the absorption of vitamin K, which helps to maintain plasma prothrombin levels. Obstruction to the flow of bile causes impaired digestion and absorption of fats, low vitamin K leading to reduced plasma prothrombin and the risk of haemorrhage. It can also cause jaundice, leading to slow healing, impairment of renal function and great risk of infection.

## NURSING CARE

Mrs Stonehouse, a 48 year old lady, is admitted to hospital to undergo cholecystectomy, accompanied by one of her two teenage daughters. She has a history of two episodes of cholecystitis in the last 6 months and has been on the waiting list for 3 months – since she saw the consultant as an out-patient. An oral cholecystogram has demonstrated the presence of gallstones in the gallbladder. Mrs Stonehouse knows of no other health problems apart from her cholecystitis.

### Pre-operative assessment
As a patient who is otherwise fit and well, Mrs Stonehouse will require routine nursing care – as laid out in the standard care plan. She was a haematologist in a London teaching hospital before her marriage and is familiar with a hospital environment which has helped her to settle in and understand what is happening.

### Potential problems
1   Possibility of bleeding during the operation.
2   Intra-abdominal infection.
3   Post-operative nausea.
4   Post-operative pain.

| NURSING ACTIONS | RATIONALE |
|---|---|
| 1   Practise good theatre aseptic technique. | Maintenance of good asepsis will avoid accidental contamination of abdominal wound. |

## NURSING ACTIONS    RATIONALE

| | |
|---|---|
| 2a) Liaise with radiographers to ensure availability at right time. | Good communications ensure that patient time on table (and under anaesthetic) is not prolonged. |
| b) Prepare operating table with X-ray translucent mattress and X-ray plates in correct situation. | Must be done in advance to allow cholangiogram without disturbing patient or contaminating sterile field. |
| c) Prepare contrast medium for the surgeon. | To ensure that correct amount of contrast medium is safely prepared and to avoid unnecessary delay. |
| 3 Anticipate surgeon's needs and supply sterile materials. | Ensures smooth operation and reduces pressure on surgeon so that he can concentrate. |
| 4a) Have diathermy equipment ready for use. b) Ensure good contact between patient and diathermy plate. c) Check patient is not touching any metal. | Diathermy used throughout operation to control minor bleeding. The current passes through the patient and must only have one path to earth – through the diathermy plate. |
| 5 Ensure that analgesia and an anti-emetic have been prescribed. | Freedom from pain and nausea during the first 24 hours will aid patient recovery. |

**Diathermy** High frequency current applied through forceps or cutting point. Tissue resistance at entry point creates enough heat to coagulate or cut. Diathermy burn is possible if the patient is in contact with any metal so current must leave patient via the diathermy plate which does not produce heat.

**The operation**

Cholecystectomy is removal of the gallbladder but often involves other procedures. The approach is usually made through a Kocher's incision – parallel to and below the lower rib on the right-hand side. Sometimes the approach is through a right upper paramedian incision (see diagram on p.45).

The incision is deepened through the layers of subcutaneous fat, abdominal muscle and peritoneum – controlling the bleeding as each layer is opened. After exploring the abdominal cavity to exclude other pathology, the surgeon retracts the liver to gain access to the gallbladder. The common bile duct is also identified and palpated for the presence of stones.

The cystic duct and artery are identified and ligated and a fine catheter is passed into the cystic duct to perform the cholangiogram. If there is any evidence of stones or obstruction the common bile duct is explored. When this has been done successfully the duct is closed around a T-tube. In addition to allowing bile drainage this enables postoperative X-rays to be taken to ensure that the bile ducts are functioning normally.

Once the surgeon is satisfied, he will remove the gallbladder which is opened to remove any obvious stones – which are usually given to the patient. The gallbladder itself is sent for histological examination. Control of bleeding from the liver after gallbladder dissection is very important so a drain will be left in situ to prevent haematoma formation or bile collection and to monitor drainage.

## Resumé of nursing actions

Mrs Stonehouse's anaesthetic was smooth and uneventful. She was then placed supine on the operating table ensuring that she was positioned so that the X-ray plates were immediately below the operative field. When anaesthetised, the patient cannot feel any sensation or move herself so care was taken that she did not sustain any pressure injuries during the operation. This was done by using support systems which spread the load on pressure points, by padding and constant awareness of the risks. Skin and tissue under pressure points, nerves and blood vessels can all be damaged by direct pressure or by shearing forces if the table is tilted. The diathermy plate can also cause undue pressure. The sacrum and heels are particularly vulnerable and pressure on the calves could increase the risk of deep vein thrombosis.

Once Mrs Stonehouse was in position, the scrub nurse assisted the surgeon to drape the patient and positioned her trolley and the Mayo table so that she could observe what the surgeon was doing and, at the same time, control the sterile instruments and supplies. She also checked that the metal of the Mayo table was not touching the patient or causing pressure on her feet.

**Mayo table**
Adjustable metal table covered with sterile drapes placed over the patient to allow easy access to sterile instruments.

The ODA working with the anaesthetist had fixed a self-adhesive diathermy plate to the right thigh and connected this to the diathermy machine. The scrub nurse now completed the diathermy circuit by handing out the end of the live diathermy cable for connection and placing the forceps in a non-conducting sterile quiver attached to the drapes. This is monopolar diathermy. You may also see bi-polar diathermy, which allows the current to pass to and from the patient via the instrument in the surgeon's hand.

The surgeon started the operation by making the skin incision. He deepened the incision through the layers of the abdominal wall and opened the peritoneal cavity. After examining the abdominal contents to confirm his diagnosis and exclude other pathology, the surgeon proceeded to dissect out the gallbladder. The scrub nurse had prepared the X-ray contrast medium (Urografin) for the cholangiogram.

**Dissection**
Separating the tissues to isolate the part to be operated on.

Urografin 150 is a radio-opaque medium used to outline the biliary tree during cholangiogram. When preparing her trolley the scrub nurse prepares a syringe with 20 ml of Urografin 150 (30%). She also prepares 20 ml of normal saline and attaches this syringe to the catheter from which she expels all the air. The surgeon inserts the catheter into the cystic duct fixing it with a ligature. He then flushes saline through the duct. The syringes are changed and Urografin injected.

It is important that no air is introduced into the biliary

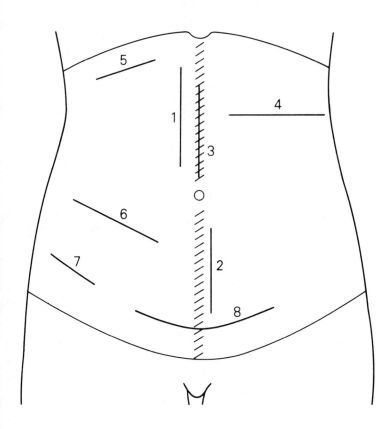

1 Right upper paramedian
2 Left lower paramedian
3 Upper midline (may be chosen for rapid access)
4 Transverse (no specific site)
5 Kocher's (for liver and gall-bladder)
6 Rutherford-Morrison (for access to iliac vessels)
7 Lanz (for appendix)
8 Pfannensteil (for pelvic operations—in the "bikini line".)

tree as the air bubbles will show up as shadows and be mistaken for stones.

Two important points for the scrub nurse are that (i) she identifies her syringes correctly and (ii) that she keeps the syringe upright above the catheter during insertion so that any air bubbles rise in the syringe and will not be injected.

The radiographers were ready to take over so after presenting the Urografin, the scrub nurse protected the wound with a sterile towel and, with the other theatre staff, retreated into the preparation room – still 'scrubbed' – leaving the anaesthetist to stop the patient's breathing for a few seconds whilst the X-rays were taken.

### X-rays of the gallbladder
*Cholecystogram (cyst=bladder)*
A diagnostic investigation in which a radio-opaque medium is taken by mouth in the form of tablets. This is concentrated in the gallbladder which then shows up as a shadow on the X-ray. Stones or polyps demonstrate as 'filling defects' in the contrast picture.

*Cholangiogram (angio=vessels)*
The contrast medium can be given intravenously or directly injected during the operation. The medium fills the biliary tree to demonstrate the patency of the biliary ducts. It also flows through into the duodenum thus demonstrating that no stone is impacted in the Ampulla of Vater. During an operative cholangiogram the patient may be tilted slightly to the right to assist the flow.

### Gallstones
Gallstones can be produced by an accumulation of fatty waste products or by precipitation of bile salts. They vary in size, number and consistency.

Once the surgeon had ensured that the cholangiogram was normal, there were no stones in the bile duct and that bile was flowing freely into the duodenum, he completed the operation, making sure that any bleeding from the liver was controlled and putting in a corrugated drain.

The scrub nurse had supplied sutures as well as checking and counting her instruments, needles and swabs throughout. She completed her duties by ensuring that the patient's

## Operative cholangiogram

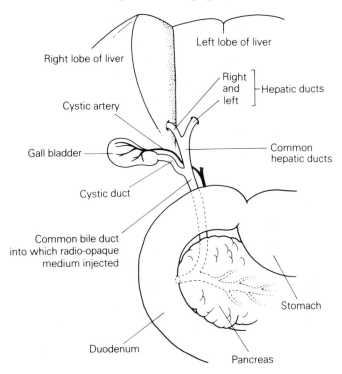

wound was clean and the dressing comfortable before she saw her patient safely off the table.

### Evaluation

Mrs Stonehouse made an uneventful recovery from the anaesthetic. Her successful recovery will be due to good theatre team work ensuring that no delay or mishap occurred during the operation. Good theatre technique enabled the surgeon to control bleeding and prevent contamination of the wound by gastro-intestinal contents. Cholecystectomy is one of the commonest operations carried out today. It is nevertheless major surgery which requires

Peritonitis

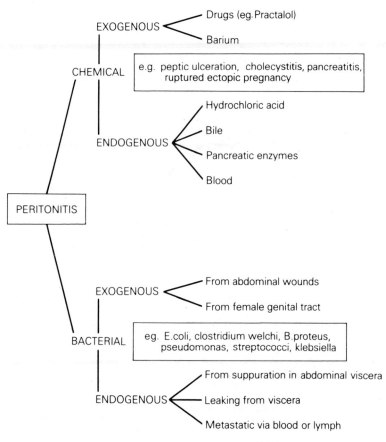

good aseptic technique to prevent unnecessary complications.

**Problems of gallbladder surgery**
1. Obstruction to the flow of bile causes the ducts to dilate.
2. A chronically inflamed gallbladder is usually thick-walled, scarred and adherent to surrounding structures.
3. The anatomy of the biliary tree is variable. The number and disposition of the ducts can vary so it is important for the surgeon to identify the various structures before tying the cystic duct. This will prevent damage to the common bile duct.

4 The arterial blood supply is also variable and must be defined to avoid tying the hepatic artery supplying the liver in mistake for the cystic artery to the gallbladder.

5 Accidental injury to the bile ducts could result in bile leaking into the peritoneal cavity causing peritonitis or a stricture of the duct and subsequent obstructive jaundice.

<table>
<tr><td>

**TEST YOURSELF**

</td><td>

1 As you read through the care plans in the book you will find a great deal of emphasis on the nurse's part in positioning the patient for surgery. Make a note of the ways in which patients are protected from injury during surgery.

</td></tr>
</table>

2 Diathermy is used in most operations.
  a) What are the correct positions for the plate?
  b) What types of diathermy plate are in use in your theatre?
  c) How do you ensure a good contact across the whole of the plate?
  Give reasons for your answers.

3 Draw a diagram of the biliary tree and label all the structures.

4 What contrast medium is used for a cholangiogram and how does the scrub nurse prepare it?

# 6 Mrs Dallas has a hysterectomy

HISTORY

Mrs Dallas is 41 years old, lives with her husband and a teenage son. She has been admitted for a total hysterectomy. She has a two-year history of heavy periods which resulted in mild anaemia for which she has been receiving iron tablets. Two months ago she had a dilation and curettage which showed that she had a small fibroid in a rather bulky uterus. In addition to this she is an asthmatic and smokes 20 cigarettes a day. She also has 'sensitive' skin and has to use special soap and make-up.

Last year her 17 year old son was killed in a road accident since when her smoking has increased and her asthma attacks have been more severe. Her obstetric history shows that she had 4 pregnancies, one was terminated and one ended in a still-birth. She is very apprehensive about the operation.

**Pre-operative anxiety** Anyone under psychological stress copes badly with physical stress. Anxious patients may 'resist' the anaesthetic thus needing more anaesthetic and beginning a spiralling situation of problems. Good emotional support and premedication help to reduce anxiety.

**Pre-operative assessment**

Mrs Dallas is presenting with a common condition requiring a straightforward operation which requires routine nursing care. She does, however, have a number of problems which could create difficulties during the anaesthetic. An anxious patient requires good nursing support. As she is a smoker as well as an asthmatic she will require good anaesthetic assessment and careful nursing observation during the recovery period.

### Anaesthetising an Asthmatic

Any asthmatic patient may present a problem for the anaesthetist because of airway problems, the risk of provoking an attack during the induction and because many asthmatics have been receiving long-term steroid therapy (e.g. prednisolone).

As long-term steroid therapy suppresses the ability of the adrenal gland to produce corticosteroids in response to the physical stress of surgery, the anaesthetist will have to give hydrocortisone cover for the period of the operation.

Mrs Dallas had not been receiving steroids but had controlled her asthma with the use of a Ventolin inhaler.

Mrs Dallas was visited pre-operatively by the theatre nurse who received her in the anaesthetic room. This had enabled the nurse to establish a relationship with Mrs Dallas, recognise her high anxiety level and give good emotional support before the operation.

**Premedication**

In view of Mrs Dallas' history the anaesthetist prescribed a premedication of pethidine and atropine to be given with aminophylline and ventolin. Pethidine is considered less likely to provoke an asthmatic response than other opiates. The aminophylline and ventolin would dilate her airways to achieve as normal a lung condition as possible.

## Problems identified

1 Anxiety due to (a) home problems
(b) fear of the operation and anaesthetic.
2 Risk of complications due to asthma and smoking.
3 Sensitive skin which could react to lotions or dressings.
4 Mild anaemia.

NURSING CARE

| NURSING ACTIONS | RATIONALE |
|---|---|
| 1 Calm confident manner with gentle precise movements. Hold Mrs Dallas' hand to give support during induction of anaesthesia. Allow her to talk if she wishes. | Good nursing support before the anaesthetic to help keep the patient's anxiety level down. |

| NURSING ACTIONS | RATIONALE |
|---|---|
| 2 Ensure that oxygen and drugs are at hand. Assist the anaesthetist to give a smooth induction. Alert the recovery nurse to problems. | Important to help ensure adequate ventilation and oxygenation to reduce risk of breathing difficulties. |
| 3 Inform surgical team so that they can use non-sensitising lotions and dressings. | To minimise the risk of allergic skin reactions. |
| 4 Ensure cross-matched blood is available in the theatre. | Ensure immediate blood replacement if there is any degree of blood loss. |

**The operation**

A total hysterectomy was carried out using a Pfannensteil incision. This is a transverse, elliptical skin incision in the fold of the skin which heals well with a good cosmetic result. The rectus sheath and peritoneum are divided using a vertical incision – the recti muscles themselves are separated and retracted. Before removing the uterus the surgeon explores the pelvis to identify structures, especially the vulnerable ureters and to exclude any other pathology.

**Ligature** A tie used for blood vessels and some other narrow vessels or pedicles.

The Fallopian tubes and ovarian ligaments are clamped, divided and ligated, preserving the ovaries. The bladder peritoneum is divided and reflected down, to allow access to the vaginal vault. The uterine artery and branches to the cervix are carefully clamped, divided and ligated. The ligaments supporting the uterus are divided and ligated and the uterus and cervix are removed. The pelvic organs are strong and muscular so gynaecological surgeons may use heavy instruments and suture with fairly thick catgut and strong needles.

The vagina and the pelvic peritoneum are closed. The abdomen is then closed in layers.

## Resumé of nursing actions

A smile and a calm manner in the anaesthetic room helped Mrs Dallas to remain relaxed. She

**Cricoid pressure (Sellick's Manoeuvre)** This means applying pressure on the larynx to push the cricoid cartilage of the larynx down onto the oesophagus. This closes the oesophagus to prevent inhalation of any regurgitated stomach contents. The pressure is not released until the endotracheal tube is in place and the cuff inflated.

**Endotracheal tube** A tube passed through the larynx into the trachea to deliver oxygen, air or anaesthetic gases.

was drowsy when she arrived but pleased to recognise the nurse and the anaesthetist. She held the nurse's hand tightly whilst she was given her injection. The nurse was prepared to apply cricoid pressure if required when the anaesthetist intubated the patient.

Once the endotracheal tube was securely in place and Mrs Dallas was stable she was moved into the operating theatre where inhalation anaesthesia was continued and an intravenous infusion of Hartmann's solution was started.

### Anaesthetic risks

Any patient with 'airway problems' will always be treated with special care by the anaesthetist. Remember that the airway to an anaesthetist is anywhere between the gas supply and the alveoli. He has to make sure that oxygen and anaesthetic gases not only get into the patient's lungs but into the blood supply and from there to the brain so all parts of the lung must be adequately inflated.

Magill cuffed and uncuffed endotracheal tubes

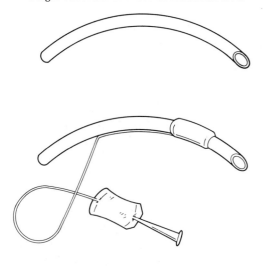

**Mrs Dallas' anaesthetic regime**

| | | |
|---|---|---|
| PREMEDICATION: | Pethidine<br>Atropine<br>Aminophylline<br>Suppository<br>+ 2 puffs<br>Ventolin | To obtain good<br>sedation and reduce<br>anxiety.<br>To obtain good<br>lung expansion<br>by dilating<br>bronchioles. |
| INDUCTION: | Methohexitone<br>Suxamethonium | An IV agent<br>Short-acting muscle<br>relaxant to paralyse<br>vocal cords and allow<br>passage of<br>endotracheal tube<br>(Intubation). |
| MAINTENANCE: | Nitrous oxide<br>Halothane<br>Oxygen | Commonly used<br>inhalation<br>anaesthetics.<br>(Halothane is a<br>broncho-dilator.) |
| | Pancuronium<br>(Pavulon) | Longer-acting<br>muscle relaxant to<br>produce relaxation of<br>the abdominal<br>muscles during the<br>operation. |
| REVERSAL: | Neostigmine | To reverse action<br>of Pavulon. |
| | Atropine | With Neostigmine –<br>to protect the heart<br>from the<br>Neostigmine which<br>can cause<br>bradycardia. |
| | Anaesthetic<br>agents | Stopped. |

Mrs Dallas' position on the table was adjusted to maintain good body alignment and prevent undue pressure on any area. Her right arm was held in place by her side and her left arm extended on an arm support to allow the anaesthetist access to the intravenous line. The diathermy plate was positioned under her left buttock ensuring good contact with the whole of the plate. Heels and calves were protected from undue pressure by the inser-

**Trendelenberg position** Used for pelvic surgery and also helps venous return from the legs and can be used if patient's blood pressure falls.

tion of a narrow pad under the achilles tendon. The table was put into a slight head down tilt (Trendelenberg) position. This allows the abdominal contents to fall back from the pelvis but not enough to embarrass the diaphragm and interfere with Mrs Dallas' breathing.

Before draping the patient the surgeon used a catheter to empty the bladder. Mrs Dallas was then prepared and draped and the Mayo table and scrub nurse's trolley positioned. The surgeon proceeded to carry out a total hysterectomy.

At the end of the operation Mrs Dallas had skin clips inserted, the vagina was swabbed out and a sterile perineal pad placed in situ.

Mrs Dallas was moved to the recovery room after her operation. The endotracheal tube had been removed and Mrs Dallas was beginning to swallow again but she was still very sleepy.

**Obstruction of the airway**
When anaesthetised, a patient is unable to guard his own airway as his swallowing and cough reflex are suppressed. He may also be paralysed and unless an endotracheal tube is in situ, we must guard the airway for the patient. We do this by supporting the jaw, inserting an artificial airway and – during recovery – by putting the patient in the left lateral position.

**Causes of obstruction**
1 Tongue falling back
2 Inhaled stomach contents
3 Laryngeal spasm.

All of these are preventable by good nursing and medical care and easily treatable if they do occur – for instance in emergency surgery.

The anaesthetist had ordered oxygen to be administered until she returned to the ward. The recovery nurse received a report on the patient from the anaesthetist and on the operation from the circulating nurse. At the same time she was supporting Mrs Dallas' jaw and observing her colour. Once she was settled into the left lateral position the recovery nurse was able to take her pulse and blood pressure and check her respiratory rate. These were recorded every 15 minutes whilst Mrs Dallas remained in the recovery room. The nurse also checked the wound and that the IV infusion was running smoothly. The second unit of Hartmann's solution was running through slowly. Mrs Dallas had not lost very much blood so none had been given although the two units were still available if they were to be needed later. Mrs Dallas stayed in the recovery room for an hour to ensure that she was breathing well and maintaining her oxygen levels. She was then settled comfortably in a clean bed before return to the ward.

**Evaluation**
Thanks to her good preparation and support pre-operatively and to a good planned anaesthetic technique, Mrs Dallas made an uneventful recovery from her anaesthetic. The surgical team had taken steps to ensure that, in addition to a good aseptic technique, they did not use any lotions or dressing materials likely to cause an allergic reaction. The major cause of anxiety about the operation had now been removed so the risk of an asthmatic attack being triggered by that anxiety was reduced. Mrs Dallas had a considerable amount of emotional stress related to her family problems and the result of her operation and needed continuing support from the ward staff.

**TEST YOURSELF**

Go and look at the ventilators in your operating theatre. Find out which type each ventilator is and ask the anaesthetist – or a member of the theatre staff who regularly works with an anaesthetist – to explain how the machine maintains the patient's ventilation.

1   What actions can a nurse take in the anaesthetic room to make a patient feel more secure?

2 Obstruction of the airway during the recovery period could be caused by –
   a) the tongue falling back
   b) vomiting
   c) laryngeal spasm.
   What action should the nurse take to prevent or treat these?

3 If Mrs Dallas had been taking long-term prednisolone, what drug would the anaesthetist have given before the operation?
   Can you explain why?

# James – a baby with congenital hypertrophic pyloric stenosis

James, a 6 week old baby, is admitted to the childrens' ward with a diagnosis of pyloric stenosis. His mother is accommodated also so that she may participate in James' care.

**Pyloric stenosis**
Congenital hypertrophic pyloric stenosis is an increase in muscle mass around the pylorus, creating a pyloric 'tumour' which obstructs the passage of milk from the stomach to the duodenum. It is four times more common in male infants than female. Signs present between two and twelve weeks of age with vomiting, which becomes projectile, towards the end of a feed or soon after. The baby may become dehydrated very quickly and lose weight or fail to thrive. On examination visible peristalsis can be observed and diagnosis is confirmed by palpation when the hypertrophied pyloric muscle can be felt. If there is any doubt, a barium meal may be performed.

James' mother will need a lot of moral support and explanation to ensure that she is fully aware of her baby's condition and the treatment planned. The doctor will explain the nature of the operation to her and obtain her consent for surgery.

She should be encouraged to participate in all aspects of James' care and can accompany him to the theatre, so maintaining close contact with him, gaining and giving reassurance.

## Pre-operative assessment

James will have special needs in the operating theatre. Such a small baby will lose body heat very rapidly, he will require careful rehydration and needs special skills in the anaesthetic room. His mother too will need a lot of support and explanation from the nursing staff.

The nurse's role in preparing James for theatre is to ensure that he is dry and warm, his intravenous infusion is progressing as ordered and the nasogastric tube is properly positioned. She should also gather the correct notes, consent forms, fluid and prescription charts and X-rays to accompany James to theatre.

Usually small babies do not require a pre-medication though Atropine 200 micrograms may be ordered to dry bronchial secretions. Paediatric drug doses are based on weight so it is important to weigh James.

| NURSING CARE | NURSING ACTIONS | RATIONALE |
|---|---|---|
| | 1 Warm theatre and heated mattress on the operating table. Incubator checked and ready. | A baby has an immature heat regulating system as well as being so small and needs extra external warmth to maintain a normal body temperature. |
| | 2 Monitor fluid intake and loss accurately to maintain adequate fluid balance. | A small baby cannot tolerate fluid loss and would quickly develop hypovolaemia if his fluid balance was not well maintained. |
| | 3 Paediatric equipment and drugs available in the theatre. | Babies are not only smaller but often anatomically and physiologically different from adults. |

| NURSING ACTIONS | RATIONALE |
|---|---|
| | Specially calibrated equipment is necessary as well as drug doses carefully measured against body weight. |
| 4 Allow mother to nurse James as much as possible. | James will gain comfort and warmth from contact with his mother but she will need support from the nurses so that she remains as calm as possible and does not feel overwhelmed by the theatre environment whilst worrying about her baby. |

**The operation**

Pyloromyotomy or Ramstedt's operation is the surgical treatment for congenital hypertrophic pyloric stenosis. A small incision is made into the upper abdomen and skin, muscle sheath and peritoneum are opened. The pylorus will be delivered through the incision by grasping with an atraumatic tissue forcep.

A small incision is made along the long axis of the pylorus. This is 'teased' open, splitting the muscle and allowing the mucosa to 'pout' out. This enlarges the lumen and allows the stomach contents to pass into the duodenum freely.

The abdominal incision is then closed in layers and a small dressing applied to the wound.

## Plan of care in reception

James arrives in reception with his mother. She is given an explanation of what is to happen to James. Care is taken to check James' identity and documents safely whilst James is nursed by his mother until the anaesthetist is ready. James's mother was well supported by the accompanying nurse so she knew what to do to help James. She was also able to feel as

## Pyloric stenosis

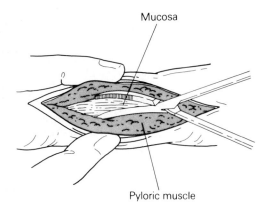

Mucosa

Pyloric muscle

comfortable as possible in this strange situation.

A small baby who is asleep in the arms of his mother or a nurse can be anaesthetised without waking him. If a mother accompanies her child into the anaesthetic room it is important for a nurse to be with her to give her the support and explanations she needs to help her child experience as little trauma as possible. The mother has to leave as soon as the child is asleep. This happens so quickly that it can be very upsetting for the mother so it is important not to forget her. She should be accompanied from the theatre by a nurse who could be ready with a comforting arm. Mothers sometimes need to be told that it is all right to cry now.

If mother – or father – does not come into the theatre it is better to say goodbye in the ward and not at the theatre door.

### In the anaesthetic room

Preparation of the anaesthetic equipment is vital for a successful operation, so every piece of equipment to be used for James has been thoroughly checked to ensure it is in working order. Suction equipment, paediatric anaesthetic equipment and paediatric doses of anaesthetic drugs are required and these have been placed ready for the anaesthetist's use.

Small babies will tolerate an inhalation induction and can be intubated without muscle relaxants. The anaesthetist monitors James' condition during the anaesthetic so an ECG (electrocardiogram), pulsometer and stethoscope are available. The nurse's role during induction of anaesthesia is to ensure James is gently restrained and kept warm. If you remember that small babies have difficulty in maintaining body heat and 80% of total body weight is fluid, the main objectives become apparent.

### Resumé of nursing actions

James is placed supine on the ready prepared heated mattress on the operating table. Care is taken to see that his limbs are in a normal position with no undue pressure on joints or nerves. Maintaining body heat is important so James' limbs and head are wrapped in gamgee.

A paediatric diathermy earth plate is placed under his buttocks. The nurse checks that the skin of the buttocks is intact and not sore and that James is not touching metal elsewhere which could offer a path to earth for the electricity generated by the use of diathermy.

### Post-operative care

Babies having this type of surgery regain consciousness very quickly. Once the operation was completed, the anaesthetist removed the endotracheal tube, ensured that James' airway was clear of any accumulated secretions and placed him on his side in the warmed incubator, ensuring a patent airway.

In recovery, the nurse maintained careful observation of James' colour, respiration, temperature and intravenous therapy. As soon as she was happy about James' condition, his mother was allowed to see him. Once fully alert with stable observations, James and his mother returned to the ward where she was able to nurse him.

Once he was fully recovered from the anaesthetic James was looking for food and he was given 30 ml of dextrose which he tolerated well.

**Evaluation**

Making the necessary adjustment to the theatre temperature, provision of a heated mattress, warm wraps and a ready prepared incubator ensured that James' temperature was kept within safe limits.

Accurate measurement of blood and fluid loss enabled the anaesthetist to replace any loss, thus maintaining hydration.

Preparation of the necessary paediatric equipment in the anaesthetic room and recovery area led to a safe uneventful anaesthetic and post-operative recovery.

Good aseptic technique reduced the risk of post-operative wound infection so James' wound should heal by first intention.

Explanation, reassurance and a kind caring attitude to James' mother went a long way in helping her overcome her anxiety.

James was able to have a successful operation in a safe environment with no post-operative complications.

TEST YOURSELF

Can you remember what it was like to be in an operating theatre for the first time? Consider what it must be like for a mother with a child about to undergo surgery. How can we support a mother so that she is herself able to give as much support as her child needs?

1  Find out the procedure in your theatre for allowing mothers to accompany their children.

2  How much blood can a small baby lose before he requires transfusion? You may find that this is much less than you expect.

# 8 Mr Wydell requires a transurethral prostatectomy

Mr Wydell is a 72 year old man who has a history of frequency and nocturia. His General Practitioner referred him to the genito-urinary consultant who has decided that Mr Wydell requires a prostatectomy as his prostate gland has become enlarged and is obstructing the outflow of urine. On examination it was discovered that Mr Wydell has a degree of hypertension and that he has chronic bronchitis.

**Hypertrophy of the prostate gland**
Many men as they grow older have some degree of prostate enlargement. It is only when this interferes seriously with the passage of urine that prostatectomy is required. Most are benign enlargements. Comparatively few men have prostate cancer and this is a slow growing cancer. Most prostate operations are carried out endoscopically as the patient is able to mobilise quickly after this. Occasionally the surgeon may carry out a **retropubic prostatectomy** and if there is pathology of the bladder as well, he may open the bladder to approach the prostate – **transvesicular prostatectomy**. Untreated prostatic enlargement can result in retention or strangury.

**Pre-operative assessment**
Mr Wydell's special nursing needs in the operating department will be related to the fact that he is an elderly man with bronchitis and hypertension. As a result of this the anaesthetist has elected to use epidural anaesthesia to reduce the respiratory risks and lower the blood pressure during the operation to help control any bleeding. Mr Wydell will need

continuous nursing support as he will be awake during his operation.

### Epidural anaesthesia
This type of anaesthesia – stricly analgesia as the patient remains awake – is known as a regional block. The analgesia affects all parts of the body supplied by the nerves which leave the spinal cord below the level of the anaesthetic. If the anaesthetist only wants to give one dose he will give it through the needle but if he wants to continue to use the epidural for the control of post-operative pain, he will pass an epidural catheter through the needle and leave this in situ taped to the patient's back to appear at shoulder level for easy access.

Some patients experience a sudden large drop in blood pressure soon after the anaesthetic is inserted. This is treated by the rapid infusion of intravenous fluids and by giving **ephedrine**. For this reason, the anaesthetist will also establish an IV line before instituting the block.

## Problems identified
1  Difficulty in breathing when lying flat.
2  Possible instability of blood pressure.
3  Anxiety during the operation.
4  Patient to be in lithotomy position during operation.
5  Post-operative bleeding leading to clot retention.
6  Possible urinary infection.

### Lithotomy position
This position is used for operations on the perineum, rectum and reproductive organs. It carries some risks unless the patient is positioned correctly.
1  The legs must be moved gently and in unison by two people to avoid the risk of hip dislocation.
2  The pelvis must remain properly supported to avoid strain on the back.
3  The legs are supported in stirrups or troughs and pressure on the calf or back of the knee must be avoided.
4  Patients with arthritis, artificial hip joints or amputations pose special problems. Sometimes a member of the theatre staff may have to support a leg during a short operation.

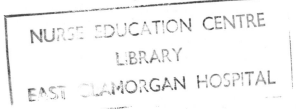

| NURSING ACTIONS | RATIONALE |
|---|---|
| 1 Retain three pillows until anaesthetic commences and allow pillows after operation. | To facilitate breathing by allowing patient to sit up except when danger of drop in blood pressure. |
| 2 Give support and explanations, assist with positioning during the epidural. Hold Mr Wydell's hand. | Assist Mr Wydell to cope with the anxiety and discomfort of the position and the procedure. |
| 3 Remain with patient to give support throughout the operation. | A patient who is awake needs support and reassurance to help him cope with the unfamiliar and stressful situation. |
| 4 Position Mr Wydell safely in lithotomy position using pads and supports. | To reduce discomfort and avoid pressure injury or joint injury. |
| 5 Observe patient and monitor blood pressure and pulse. | The patient is normally hypertensive but is to be given an epidural which will lower his blood pressure. |
| 6 Monitor urinary drainage. | To recognise post-operative bleeding or clot retention which may require a bladder washout. |

## NURSING ACTIONS  RATIONALE

7  Practise good          To prevent ascending
   aseptic technique      urinary infection.
   when dealing with
   catheter and
   urinary drainage
   system.

### The operation

Strictly speaking this operation should be termed
'per-urethral' and that may be the term used in your
theatre. The operation is carried out using a **resectoscope**.
This is a modification of a **cystoscope** which allows:

a) passage of irrigation fluid to dilate the bladder.
b) passage of a diathermy loop electrode to resect away
   the prostate gland.
c) visualisation of the operative site by the use of a
   telescope and fibre-optics.

The surgeon first of all examines the prostate gland and
bladder to establish the extent of any pathology. He then
inserts the loop electrode. The resectoscope has a trigger
which allows the surgeon to pull the loop through that
part of the prostate gland which is occluding the urethra
until he has established an unobstructed pathway
through the gland. He can also touch the diathermy
electrode onto small bleeding points to obtain
haemostasis (i.e. stop the bleeding!). All this is observed
by the surgeon who views the site through the telescope.

Light is provided along a flexible fibre-optic cable from
a light-box. As the small pieces of resected prostate gland
collect within the bladder they are washed out by the
use of an **evacuator**. They are collected in a sieve by the
scrub nurse and sent to the laboratory for a histology
report. The surgeon takes great care not to damage the
internal urethral sphincter so that the patient will
remain continent; or to traumatise the urethral wall
which could cause stricture.

## In the anaesthetic room

Equipment for intravenous fluids and a sterile
trolley with epidural equipment were ready in
the anaesthetic room when Mr Wydell arrived.
His theatre nurse received him into her care
from the ward nurse and explained with the
anaesthetist what was to happen.

### Drugs used for epidural anaesthesia
*Bupivacaine (Marcaine)*
Probably the most commonly used, this is a long-acting agent and works for about 4–6 hours.
*Lignocaine*
Shorter acting local anaesthetic.
*Morphine + Methadone*
These opiates can also be instilled for longer-acting pain control. Methadone is used to treat post-operative pain after caesarian section. Morphine is used in a similar way and both drugs are useful in the treatment of intractable cancer pain. A much smaller dose than the standard IM injection gives good pain control for a longer period of time.

An IV infusion of normal saline was commenced before Mr Wydell was turned into the left lateral position. The anaesthetist then commenced the epidural injection using full aseptic technique. After the anaesthetist was satisfied that analgesia had been established satisfactorily, Mr Wydell was settled with one pillow, given an injection of Diazemuls and positioned in the lithotomy position with his legs in Lloyd Davis troughs. He was then wheeled into theatre.

### Resumé of nursing actions
The nurse stayed by him to give verbal support and monitor his condition for the anaesthetist. An anaesthetic screen was used to raise the table drapes off Mr Wydell's face. An electronic monitor was used to monitor Mr Wydell's pulse, ECG and blood pressure continuously. He was now very sleepy though he held on to the nurse's hand for most of the operation and was able to respond to questions. Everyone in theatre was careful about their conversation as they were aware that Mr Wydell was awake.

At the end of the operation the surgeon inserted a three-way catheter and established continuous bladder drainage. The scrub nurse made sure that Mr Wydell was clean and dry. The nurse explained what was happening and alerted Mr Wydell as his legs were lowered and he was repositioned on the table before he was lifted back onto his bed.

**In the recovery ward**
Mr Wydell's nurse accompanied him to the recovery ward. His urinary drainage was running freely. It was heavily blood-stained at first but there was no sign of clot retention as the catheter was draining freely. Blood pressure was checked every 15 minutes and as it remained stable Mr Wydell was allowed three pillows and returned to the ward after about 45 minutes in recovery.

**Evaluation**
Mr Wydell had been assessed pre-operatively by the anaesthetist who elected to avoid a general anaesthetic as this would be more of a risk for the patient. It is an advantage to use an epidural for a hypertensive patient, as it lowers blood pressure and may help to reduce bleeding both during and after the operation. Good support by a nurse specially delegated to care for Mr Wydell helped him cope with the stress of being awake during the operation and allowed the nurse to monitor his condition and assist the anaesthetist if his blood pressure had fallen sharply.

This is a common but necessary operation in an age group which has a high incidence of medical problems similar to Mr Wydell's.

TEST
YOURSELF

1 Ask to be shown the instruments required for transurethral resection and practise setting up the irrigation fluid.

2 List the equipment and drugs laid up for an epidural anaesthesia in your theatre.

3 a) Look up the anatomy of the prostate gland.
   b) Define *strangury*.

c) What are the symptoms of prostatism?
d) Does some understanding of the procedures help you in caring for someone with this condition? How?

4  Mr Wydell was given diazepam.
   a) Why was this?
   b) How was this administered?
   c) What dosage did the anaesthetist give?
   d) What are the dangers?

# 9    Mrs Mann has a laparoscopy

HISTORY

Mrs Mann, aged 26, is to be admitted as a day patient for laparoscopic examination. She has a history of pelvic pain and dyspareunia which her General Practitioner has diagnosed as being due to an ovarian cyst, but no evidence of this was found during an outpatient clinic examination two days ago. It has therefore been decided to admit her for laparoscopy.

## Pre-operative assessment

During her outpatient visit, Mrs Mann was carefully medically assessed to ensure her fitness to undergo surgery under general anaesthetic and to be discharged home the same day.

This medical assessment shows her to be a fit young lady with no history of respiratory problems and no recent colds and so it has been decided she is suitable for day surgery. She has no stiffness of hips or knees which could cause problems during positioning on the operating table for laparoscopy.

Mrs Mann has been given written instructions about her preparation at home and these were explained to her by the nurse so that she fully understands the importance of fasting from midnight on the night prior to admission. The nurse also explained to Mrs Mann that after the general anaesthetic, she would not be able to drive so that she should arrange for her husband to bring her and collect her once she was ready for discharge home.

### Day surgery

Day surgery is only suitable for individuals who are fit. Anyone with a history of cardiac or respiratory problems or who has had an adverse reaction to general

71

anaesthetic in the past is not considered for day case surgery and requires to be admitted for a longer period post-operatively to ensure complications do not develop.

Mrs Mann is to arrive on the day ward two hours prior to the operation and her preparation includes:

1 Checking documentation details including consent for surgery and anaesthetic which had been obtained during her outpatient visit.
2 Application of identity wrist band.
3 Changing into theatre gown.
4 Continuing the fast begun at home.
5 Allowing her to rest quietly in bed.

As Mrs Mann appears relaxed about the procedure, no premedication has been ordered and she is left to rest quietly once all routine pre-operative preparation has been carried out.

She is transferred from the ward to theatre on a trolley accompanied by a ward nurse.

## NURSING CARE

| NURSING ACTIONS | RATIONALE |
|---|---|
| 1 Preserve a quiet environment. | No premedication has been given therefore patient is fully aware of surroundings. |
| 2 Preserve dignity by avoiding undue exposure especially whilst awake. | Position for operation means removal of some covers. |
| 3 Have all table attachments ready – lithotomy poles and shoulder rests. | Prevents prolonging anaesthetic. |

## NURSING ACTIONS   RATIONALE

4   Care when            Prevents sciatic
    adopting lithotomy   nerve damage.
    position. Raise
    both legs together.
    LIFT buttocks to     Prevents strain on
    end of table         nerves and muscles
    but ensure           of hip joints and
    well supported.      lower back.
    Check position of    Prevents pressure
    legs against         on calves.
    lithotomy poles.
    On completion        Prevents sciatic
    lower legs           nerve damage.
    together.

5   Recover in           Prevents airway
    lateral position     obstruction.
    on completion
    until conscious.

**Laparoscopy**
Laparoscopy is a procedure which enables the surgeon to
inspect the pelvic organs, take biopsy of tissue and carry
out certain operations through an endoscope.

The patient is placed in the lithotomy position once
anaesthetised. The urinary bladder is emptied via a
catheter and a bi-manual examination of the pelvic
region undertaken.

The vulval region and the abdomen, having been
shaved in the ward, are cleaned with antiseptic solution.
The surgeon uses a solution with an aqueous base for the
vulval area as this is less traumatic to sensitive tissues.
The abdomen is covered with sterile towels and the legs
are covered with sterile leggings.

The cervix is grasped by a vulsellum forceps, the uterus
is curetted and a speculum or sound placed in the cervix.
This allows the surgeon, or an assistant, to move the
uterus about during the procedure. The table is tilted to
allow the abdominal contents to fall away from the pelvis
and about 4 litres of $CO_2$ are inserted into the peritoneal
cavity through a cannula.

A small incision is made just below the umbilicus and
a trocar and cannula wide enough to accommodate a
laparoscope are inserted into the space created by the $CO_2$.
Visual examination of the pelvic structures is carried
out through this laparoscope. Biopsies or laparoscopic

sterilisation can be carried out using a second cannula whilst the surgeon maintains direct vision through the laparoscope.

On completion of the procedure, as much of the carbon dioxide as possible is expelled from the abdomen. The abdominal incision is closed either by skin tapes, clips or sutures which can usually be removed 2–3 days after the investigation.

Patients may complain of shoulder tip pain following this procedure. This is referred pain from the diaphragm, caused by the distension of the abdomen by the carbon dioxide. Explanation of the cause of this and oral analgesia are usually all that is required, as the carbon dioxide is reabsorbed by the peritoneum.

## Resumé of nursing actions

Mrs Mann is transferred from the trolley to lie in the dorsal position on the full operating table until the general anaesthetic has been induced. The operating table is one on which the foot end of the table can be detached to allow the surgeon easier access to work in the perineal area once the patient is in the lithotomy position.

Mrs Mann's anaesthetic is induced using Sodium Thiopentone 250 mg and Atracurium 25 mg via a needle placed in a vein in the back of her hand. An endotracheal tube is passed and connected to a Manley ventilator and anaesthetic maintained with nitrous oxide and oxygen.

### Artificial ventilation

Any paralysed patient is obviously unable to breathe for him or herself. Every theatre will have at least one, sometimes several, ventilators of one type or another. All of them work by pumping oxygen and gases into the lungs (inspiratory phase) then tripping a switch (cycling) to stop the pump. This allows the patient's lungs to collapse and the patient breathes out (expiratory phase).

During induction a nurse in the anaesthetic room gives Mrs Mann support and reassurance.

Once settled on the ventilator in theatre, Mrs Mann is moved into the lithotomy position, care being taken to elevate both legs together to avoid back strain and sciatic nerve damage. Care is also taken to lift her buttocks over the end of the table in order to avoid damage to skin in the sacral area through friction. The table is then tilted head-down into the Trendelenberg position. Mrs Mann is now ready for the surgeon to carry out laparoscopy.

Lithotomy position

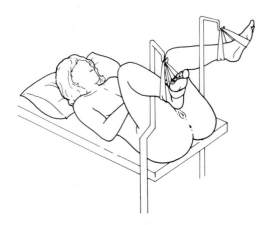

On completion of the examination Mrs Mann's legs are lifted down from the lithotomy poles together, the anaesthetist carefully removes the endotracheal tube and places an oral airway in position before turning her into the left lateral position to recover and regain her cough and swallow reflex.

Mrs Mann is then returned to the ward to rest quietly in bed and she will be discharged home when her husband collects her in the early evening.

She will be reminded not to drive during the next few days until the effects of the general anaesthetic have been completely eliminated from her body.

1 What type of drug is Sodium Thiopentone and how does it act?

2 Why was Mrs Mann given Atracurium along with Sodium Thiopentone during induction of anaesthetic?

3 For what reason may the operating table be tipped into the Trendelenburg position during laparoscopy?

4 Describe what you understand by the term bi-manual examination.

5 Which nerve pathway transmits the referred pain from the diaphragm to the shoulder tip?

# 10 Mrs White is admitted for a bronchoscopy

Mrs White, aged 51 years, has been admitted to a thoracic surgical ward for an investigative bronchoscopy. She has been referred by her General Practitioner following a period of increasing breathlessness on exertion and because of an area of opacity in the lower lobe of the left lung on a recent chest X-ray.

Mrs White is a non-smoker and is otherwise in good health.

**Bronchoscopy is necessary to assist in making a diagnosis**
1. Biopsy of tissue from the area of opacity will be sent for laboratory examination – cytology.
2. Aspirated bronchial secretions will be examined for culture and sensitivity of organisms.
3. Aspirated bronchial secretions will be examined for presence of abnormal cells.

## Pre-operative assessment

Mrs White is admitted on the day prior to the bronchoscopy so that pre-operative preparation can be carried out, which includes information about her nursing needs.

| | |
|---|---|
| 1 Collection of nursing data: | |
| a) Information about dentition. | Loose or capped teeth are at risk; bronchoscope is passed orally. |
| b) Information about neck stiffness. | Hyperextension of neck is necessary to pass rigid bronchoscope. |
| 2 Arrange for chest X-rays and tomography. | To detect any changes since previous X-rays. |

| 3 | Introduce deep breathing exercises. | Improve oxygenation and aid expectoration post-operatively. |
| 4 | Listen to any worries expressed and give information to reduce anxiety. | Possible fears of malignancy. |

Routine preparation as for any operation under general anaesthetic is carried out and Mrs White has been warned that she may experience some discomfort in her throat and neck following the examination due to the passing of the endoscope and the position of her head whilst the procedure is carried out. She is also told that she may cough up a little blood-stained sputum afterwards if a biopsy of tissue is taken, and that this soon stops so she need not be alarmed.

Transfer from ward to theatre on a trolley with stretcher canvas and poles. This is to enable an easy return to the trolley on completion of the bronchoscopy whilst Mrs White is still unconscious.

**A suggestion**
If there is an operating table in your theatre which is used for bronchoscopy, try lying on it for a few minutes and experience the feelings the patient is likely to have as she awaits the induction of her anaesthetic. Note how vulnerable you may feel, the position your legs adopt and how little room there is for your arms.

Beware – do be careful with your head and neck – have a colleague with you for safety!

| NURSING CARE | NURSING ACTIONS | RATIONALE |
| --- | --- | --- |
| | 1 Correct positioning of the table. Care with head and neck on small headrest. | Head could become unsupported. |

| | | |
|---|---|---|
| 2 | Ensure eyes are closed after induction. | Prevent corneal damage. |
| 3 | Care to retain arms safely. | Prevent ulnar nerve injury. |
| 4 | Ensure legs are uncrossed once anaesthetised. | Prevent pressure on calves and achilles tendons. |
| 5 | On completion of bronchoscopy turn onto left side. | Allows unaffected lung to expand to maximum. |
| 6 | Ensure oral airway is in position until cough and swallow reflex return. | |
| 7 | Observe for signs of stridor indicated by noisy breathing. | Prevent airway obstruction. |
| 8 | Keep mouth clear of secretions, sputum or blood from biopsy. | |
| 9 | Monitor pulse and respiration frequently until conscious. | Detect any change in condition. |

**Bronchoscopy**

This is a procedure which may be carried out under general or local anaesthetic. There are also flexible fibre-optic bronchoscopes available in some theatre units. Visual inspection, collection of secretions and biopsy of tissue are possible during the examination.

An effective means of applying suction down the bronchoscope is necessary and a means of giving oxygen down the bronchoscope is vital as the patient is unable to breath during the procedure as muscle relaxant drugs are given to enable the surgeon to pass the endoscope.

A number of metal suction tubes are available, with

malleable gum elastic tips which can be angled to pass into branches of the bronchi in case any one becomes blocked.

A Luken sputum trap can be added into the suction connecting tubing in order to collect bronchial secretion specimens.

Luken sputum trap

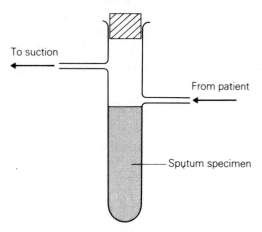

*Tissue biopsy forceps* – straight and angled are required to obtain biopsies from various bronchial branches.
*Direct, right-angled and retrograde viewing telescopes* may also be used to enable a better view of bronchi.
Although usually a very short procedure, bronchoscopy is not without risks.

### Resumé of nursing actions

Two nurses will be involved during the bronchoscopy, one to look after Mrs White's care and the other to handle the bronchoscopy equipment.

Mrs White is received into theatre having been prepared for general anaesthetic and given a premedication of Papaveretum 10 mg and Scopolamine 0.2 mg by intramuscular injection one hour previously to alleviate anxiety and reduce salivary secretions which could pass into the lungs whilst she is unconscious.

Great care is taken in positioning Mrs White's head on the small headrest as the surgeon is using a rigid bronchoscope, which means the neck will have to be extended sufficiently to bring the mouth into alignment with the trachea and bronchi during the examination. Mrs White's left arm is supported at a comfortable angle on an arm rest to give the anaesthetist access for intravenous anaesthetic drugs. Her right arm is supported by her side; one of the nurses is delegated to monitor her radial pulse throughout the procedure. All these actions are explained to Mrs White as they are carried out before she is given her anaesthetic injection.

A dressing towel is placed under her head in readiness to cover the eyes and hair once Mrs White is anaesthetised.

As the endoscope is passed via the mouth it is necessary to ensure the eyes are closed and covered by a towel to prevent damage, as the outer end of the endoscope is in close proximity to the eyes during the procedure.

Care to prevent damage to the front teeth by the bronchoscope is needed and for this reason the surgeon may protect them with gauze swabs.

Once in control of her cough and swallow reflex, Mrs White can be returned on the trolley to the ward. She should initially be encouraged to lie on the side from which biopsy has been taken as this allows the unaffected lung to expand fully and give good oxygenation. Should Mrs White suffer from a sore throat or neck afterwards, analgesia may need to be prescribed and given.

The patient's **radial pulse** will be continuously monitored and any change reported to the anaesthetist. As the patient is not breathing, she can quickly become hypoxic if oxygen is not passed into the lungs intermittently during the procedure.

TEST YOURSELF

Find out how local anaesthetic is used for bronchoscopy and what special precautions are needed before and after its use.

Ask sister or staff nurse to show you the type of equipment available in your theatre for carrying out bronchoscopy.

Try to be present when a bronchoscopy is

done – the surgeon may let you have a look down the bronchoscope.

1   In cases of suspected lung disease, other diagnostic procedures may be carried out. Define the following:
    Bronchography
    Tomography.

2   Do you know what is meant by Vital Capacity and Forced Expiratory Volume?

3   What does the term stridor mean and should it arise, what nursing action would be taken to relieve it?

# Simon needs correction of strabismus

11

Simon, who is 3 years old, has been admitted for correction of strabismus. His mother had noticed that Simon had a 'squint' and had taken him to the General Practitioner who referred him to the Ophthalmic Surgeon. For 18 months Simon has been attending Ophthalmic Outpatients in an attempt to correct the squint by conservative means. The surgeon has now decided that surgery is necessary to correct the deviation of the eye by resecting the right lateral rectus muscle of the right eye.

### Physiology

| *Normal* | *Abnormal* |
|---|---|
| In the human, both eyes fixate on one object to produce binocular single vision. The light rays enter each pupil and are refracted to corresponding points on each retina. As objects move closer the eyes converge to maintain fixation and hence a single image. This is brought about by the co-ordinated action of the extrinsic eye muscles. | In a squint, binocular single vision has been lost and the eye deviates as a result of one muscle, usually the medial rectus but sometimes the lateral rectus, being stronger than its antagonist. Whilst one eye fixates on the object, the other eye appears to be fixated on a different object which can lead to diplopia and later monocular vision if amblyopia (laziness) develops. |

Simon's father is a sales representative and is frequently away from home and he has an 8 year old sister who is at a primary school close to the hospital. This means that his mother will not be able to stay with Simon throughout his stay in hospital.

On admission at 10 o'clock in the morning,

Simon is accompanied by his mother and Bruno, his favourite teddy bear who will stay with him!

## Pre-operative assessment

Although Simon is apparently at ease in the hospital following his regular visits as an out-patient, he has never been away from home on his own before. This is a frightening experience for a three year old who is to be exposed to strange, not to say awe-inspiring, experiences when he comes to the operating theatre. His mother may also feel anxious and guilty that she is unable to stay with him. Eye surgery is precise and demanding so the theatre and equipment must be prepared and used with care. The anaesthetic team will have prepared paediatric equipment and drug doses will be estimated against Simon's small body weight.

### Paediatric anaesthesia

Small children are rarely given an intravenous anaesthetic as childrens' veins are small and it is a frightening and painful experience for a child. It is more usual to give inhalation anaesthesia. Once the child is asleep the anaesthetist will insert a butterfly needle so that he has an open vein for any other drugs he may wish to give. This is done very quickly. **Suxamethonium** – a rapid acting muscle relaxant – can then be given to relax the vocal cords to allow passage of an endotracheal tube.

All drug doses for children are scaled down according to their body weight.

## Problems identified

1  Simon will be frightened unless given loving and understanding care.
2  Mother may be unduly anxious unless well supported.

**NURSING CARE**

| NURSING ACTIONS | RATIONALE |
|---|---|
| 1  Allow mother to stay with Simon until he is anaesthetised. Also allow Bruno to remain with him. | Simon will need his mother's support and the presence of a familiar toy will help him cope with his fear and uncertainty. |

| NURSING ACTIONS | RATIONALE |
|---|---|
| 2 Allow role play with equipment. Encourage Simon to blow up the (reservoir bag) balloon before turning on the anaesthetic gases. Do not force Simon to lie down if he doesn't want to. Mother or nurse can cuddle him and he can be anaesthetised sitting up on mum's lap. | Ideally the nurse would visit Simon on the ward and allow the role play there so that he would meet a familiar face and recognise something he had played with and knew how to use. |
| 3 Explain the operation and preparation to mother – and what she will be able to do to help Simon. | Mother needs explanation and support so that she can hold and help Simon without feeling overwhelmed or lost in a strange environment. |
| 4 Encourage mother to stay as long as she can – at least until Simon wakes up – and to leave Bruno with him. | Simon will find it difficult to understand why mother has left and could feel rejected or punished by her absence. Bruno can be the family representative with him. |
| 5 Ensure body weight is accurately recorded. | To prevent risk of drug overdose. |

**Reservoir bag**
Large rubber bag included in an anaesthetic circuit to allow mixing of gases. The bag reduces turbulence in the gas flow and ensures an even flow without changes of pressure inside the circuit.

## NURSING ACTIONS    RATIONALE

**Headring**  Used to
prevent the head
moving from side
to side as pressure
is applied during
surgery.

6  Ensure that
   paediatric
   headring is
   available in the
   theatre.

To ensure stability of
the head during
surgery.

7  Instill antibiotic
   eye-drops as
   prescribed,
   checking the
   bottle with the
   surgeon prior to
   installation.

To minimise the risk
of infection.

**Speculum**
Instrument for
retracting the
eyelids. Held in
place by pressure of
the instrument
against
counter-pressure of
the eyelid, allowing
easy access to the
underlying
structures of the
eye.

**The operation**
Lateral rectus resection involves the resection of a length
of lateral eye muscle thus allowing the eyeball to return
to its normal central axis enabling single binocular vision
to be resumed.

After preparing the skin with a suitable cleansing
lotion and draping the head, the surgeon makes his first
incision. The eyelids are held apart by a speculum or stay
suture to allow an incision through the conjunctiva to
expose the lateral muscle which is to be resected. The
point of origin is established and the muscle is measured
using calipers which are then set to allow a check after
the muscle has been resected. After resection the
conjunctiva is sutured using very fine absorbable sutures.

### In the anaesthetic room

As Simon was only admitted on the morning
of surgery, it was not possible to visit him on
the ward pre-operatively but the ward nurses
had given explanations to his mother who
accompanied him into the anaesthetic room.

She was able to sit on a specially provided
chair in the anaesthetic room with Simon on
her lap cuddling Bruno. The anaesthetist made
a game of giving the anaesthetic, allowing
Simon to blow into the balloon which he did
with some apprehension, eventually falling
asleep on his mother's knee. He was then lifted
onto the operating table and induction of
anaesthesia was completed whilst his mother

Recti of the left eye

1 Superior rectus        4 Inferior rectus
2 Medial rectus          5 Inferior oblique
3 Lateral rectus         6 Superior oblique

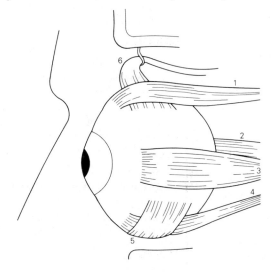

was accompanied out to the recovery ward to await his arrival.

**Resumé of nursing actions**
Simon was positioned on the table with his head secured in the headring near the top of the table and he was draped ready for surgery. After the eyelids had been retracted by a speculum the conjunctiva was incised and the muscle exposed. The muscle was shortened after exact measurement with calipers to ensure that the eye deviation was not overcorrected. After the conjunctiva had been repaired antibiotic eyedrops were instilled and following extubation, Simon was transferred to a theatre trolley with safety rails.

### In the recovery ward

Simon had been placed on his right side and Bruno was placed at his side so that he was the first thing Simon saw as he woke up. Pulse and respiration were observed every fifteen minutes and his mother was allowed to sit by his side.

As Simon's condition was satisfactory he was escorted back to the ward by the nurse and his mother after thirty minutes.

Simon's mother had to leave him after he fell asleep in the ward but she returned to take him home the following morning. She was then shown how to instill the eyedrops before taking Simon and Bruno home.

### Evaluation

Hopefully Simon will have learned to be unafraid of hospitals and anaesthetics, as he was well supported throughout and did not feel abandoned by his mother.

| TEST YOURSELF |
| --- |

1 Draw and label a diagram of both eyes. Label all the external muscles of both eyes.

2 What other treatment may Simon have received prior to surgery? Name the personnel who will have been involved in this treatment.

3 Explain what is meant by:
   a) divergent squint
   b) convergent squint.

# 12 The other side of the coin

The patient in the operating department is, as we have seen, very physically dependent on the medical and nursing staff who are caring for him. For the surgeon and anaesthetist this is an awesome responsibility as, during the operation, they may have to take away even the patient's ability to support his own respiration and circulation. **No operation can be without risk.** The need for surgery must be carefully weighed against the patient's condition and his ability to withstand the stress of surgery. Surgery can in some ways be regarded as a failure of medicine. If medicine cannot cure, it may be possible to repair, bypass or replace an organ or a limb by surgical intervention.

To operate successfully, the surgeon must concentrate on the operation itself, delegating the general care of the patient to the anaesthetist and the nursing staff.

We hope that during your stay in theatre you will gain valuable insights into the work of the theatre team but more particularly, into your patients' experiences whilst undergoing surgery and anaesthesia.

It is very easy to forget that what is routine for the nursing staff may be a **major life event** for the patient. Can you imagine the stress on a woman who has discovered a lump in her breast, who goes to her doctor and is rapidly admitted to hospital? On admission she is asked to consent to an operation which carries the possibility of her waking up to find that her breast has been removed, confirming her worst fears that she has cancer. We may know that the vast majority of breast lumps are benign, as we see many of these operations, but nearly every one of these women has been exposed to the possibility that the operation may proceed to mastectomy.

Many operations are routine and the patient knows friends and family members who have recovered rapidly and successfully. Others are mutilating operations with far-reaching effects on the patient's life and ability to carry on as before. They may require intensive nursing care in hospital and will have to modify their lives to cope with the result of the operation. Some of these operations, such as mastectomy, damage the patient's **self-image**. Some require counselling and education to be able to live with the results afterwards. An elderly patient with a colostomy or joint replacement may find the pre-operative explanations so confusing and stressful that they abdicate any control of their life to us and put a great deal of trust in our care during the traumatic experience which they are undergoing.

A person's fear of the unknown – and fear of how he or she will react to pain and dependency – will increase anxiety and require good support from both ward and theatre staff.

We could define the **ideal patient** as one who has one illness for which he requires surgery but is otherwise fit. Now that we are operating increasingly on elderly people, we see more patients who have other illnesses to complicate the picture. Mrs Dallas was an asthmatic; Mr Wydell had bronchitis and hypertension. Some patients may never have slept away from home or shared a bedroom, never mind being exposed to some of the more intimate and distressing procedures involved in the preparation and procedures of modern surgery.

A problem-solving approach to nursing helps to identify some of these psychosocial needs and to plan the necessary care.

Good explanations and support depend on good **communications**. The patient may find difficulty in expressing his worries so nurses should learn to become more aware of the non-verbal signs of stress and anxiety. This is particularly important in the anaesthetic room, where the theatre nurse may have very little time to establish a rapport with the patient who may be sleepy and want to stay that way. On the other hand he may have a great need to talk. It is very important for patients who are deaf or partially sighted to retain their hearing aid or glasses until they are anaesthetised. There is no right or wrong thing to say but a smile, using the patient's name and holding his hand will tell him that you are aware that he is very anxious and that you are there to support him.

Finally, we should remember the importance of allowing the patient to rest quietly and, if possible, sleep after his premedication. He will be disturbed by being transported to theatre but a long wait after arrival in theatre or suddenly finding that he has not signed a consent form can be very distressing and will only contribute to already considerable anxiety.

Try not to let your own anxiety in a new environment or fear of doing the wrong thing interfere with your ability to recognise the patient's needs. Your worry about working in a strange environment like theatre can be a valuable experience to help you understand some of your patient's feelings.

# 13 Writing a care study

When you come to work in theatre it is sometimes difficult to get the total picture of what is happening to the patient. Unless you visit the patient on the ward pre- and post-operatively and then both receive and recover the patient as well as accompanying him into theatre, you will only see a part of what happens. As a learner you may be allowed to do just that with at least one patient and may then be expected to write a care study.

Writing a care study, as you probably are aware, is rather different from writing a care plan. You will need to include all the details in the standard care plan (pp. 35–40), as well as the plans for the individual problems of that patient.

Using a problem-solving approach to planning nursing care requires a framework of concepts about the patient, about nursing and about the aims of care – in short, a model of nursing. Within the limits of a model you can assess the patient's degree of ill-health, his need for nursing intervention and the goals of your nursing action. Is the patient capable of carrying out his activities of daily living (Roper Logan & Tierney)? What is his ability for self care (Orem)? How is the patient adapting to stress (Saxton & Hyland)?

We will look at the stages of planning nursing care using several different models for the different stages of the process.

1   Assessing the patient (using Roper)

a)   How old is the patient?
How does this affect the degree of independence which we can expect of this patient when he is not undergoing surgery?

A baby or a very elderly and frail patient will be much more dependent than a strapping young rugby player!

The difference between normal independence and the degree of dependence experienced by the patient coming to theatre can influence the patient's reaction to losing control of his life – even for a very short time.

b)   Next, you might consider each Activity of Living (AL)

1   on arrival in theatre
2   on the operating table
3   on arrival in the recovery ward
4   on leaving the recovery ward.

Plot these in different coloured inks on the Roper model diagram and it will demonstrate quite dramatically how a patient moves to a condition of total dependence in the middle of an operation if he has been given a general anaesthetic. You might like to compare this with the different situation for a patient undergoing surgery using a local analgesic.

## The Roper, Logan & Tierney model of nursing

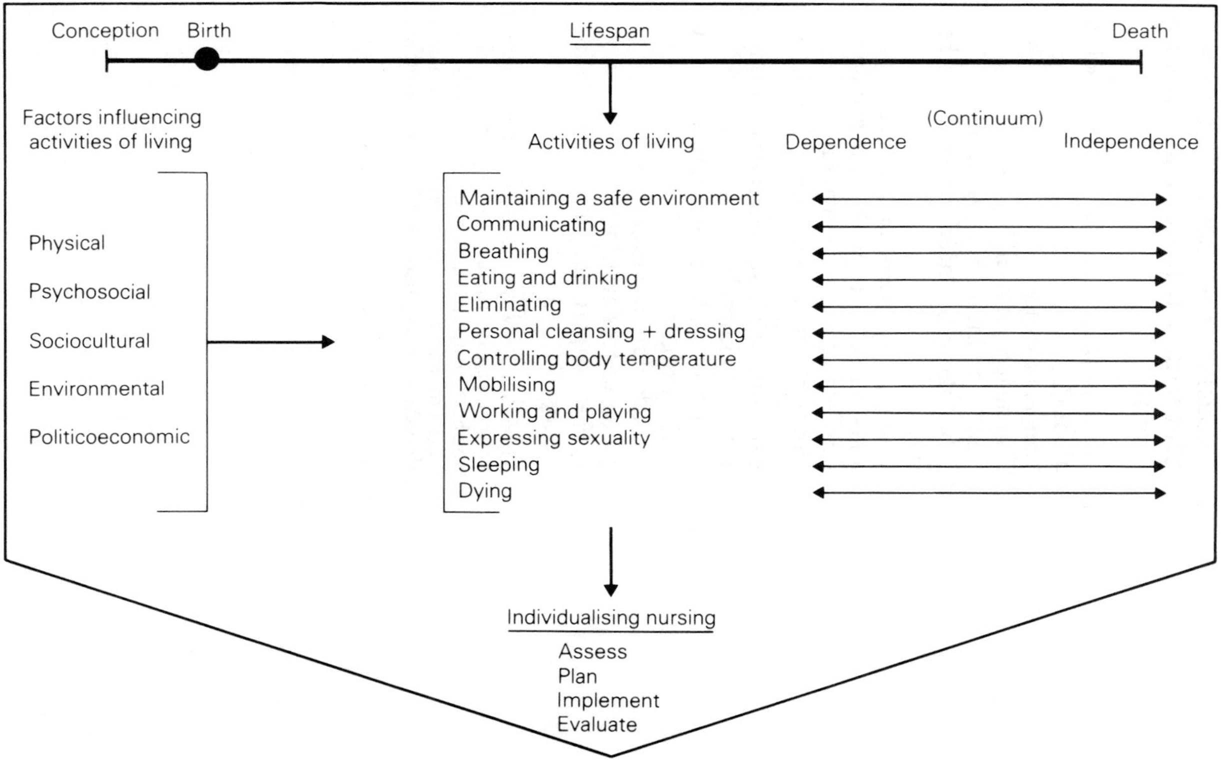

2  Identifying the patient's needs and problems while in theatre (using Orem)

a) What is the patient's deficit in self-care ability?
Can he breathe?
Can he feed himself?
Can he maintain his fluid intake?
What about his need for rest or to be active?
Compare his need for solitude or privacy and his need to be with other people.
Can he maintain his own safety?
How far is he from his normal (well) state?

b) Does this self-care deficit result from:
   1 Lack of knowledge
   2 Lack of skills or strength to deal with the situation
   3 Lack of motivation
   4 Age or present illness
   5 Past experience affecting ability to 'cope'?

This is another way to assess the patient's needs. If you compare the two approaches you will find that you have identified very similar problems but one model may be more appropriate to your patient than the other – or they may complement each other.

Orem's self care model of nursing

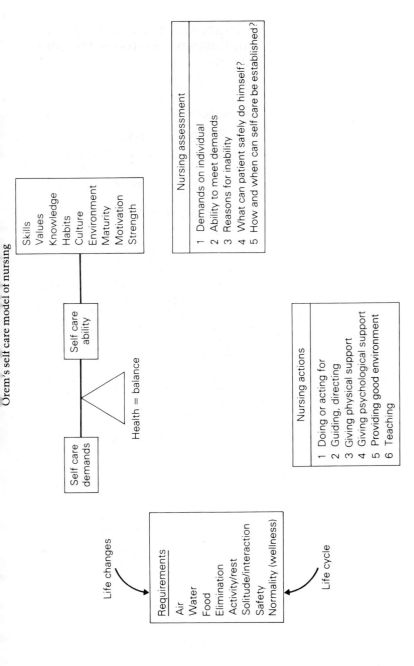

## 3 Consider the factors which affect your patient (Saxton & Hyland)

Are they mainly:

a) physical factors or
b) psychological factors.

Using the Saxton and Hyland Nursing Assessment Graph it is possible to identify whether the priority needs for nursing care are in the physiological or psychological area. For example:

Patient with subdural haematoma

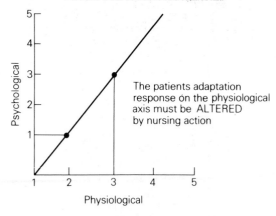

The patients adaptation response on the physiological axis must be ALTERED by nursing action

Patient with possible mastectomy

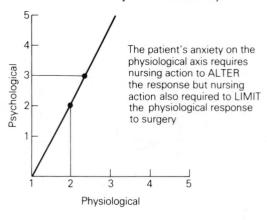

The patient's anxiety on the physiological axis requires nursing action to ALTER the response but nursing action also required to LIMIT the physiological response to surgery

## Saxton & Hyland stress adaptation model of nursing

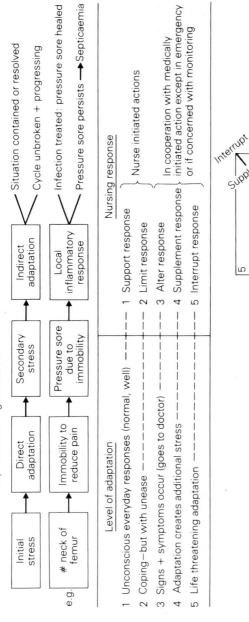

Stress = ∨ Primary stressors – local
         ∨ Secondary stressors – generalised

| Initial stress | → | Direct adaptation | → | Secondary stress | → | Indirect adaptation | → | Situation contained or resolved / Cycle unbroken + progressing |

e.g. # neck of femur → Immobility to reduce pain → Pressure sore due to immobility → Local inflammatory response → Infection treated: pressure sore healed / Pressure sore persists → Septicaemia

### Level of adaptation

1 Unconscious everyday responses (normal, well) - - - - - - 1 Support response
2 Coping – but with unease - - - - - - - - - - - - - - - 2 Limit response
3 Signs + symptoms occur (goes to doctor) - - - - - - - - 3 Alter response
4 Adaptation creates additional stress - - - - - - - - - - 4 Supplement response
5 Life threatening adaptation - - - - - - - - - - - - - - 5 Interrupt response

### Nursing response

1 Support response ⎫
2 Limit response    ⎬ Nurse initiated actions
3 Alter response   ⎭
4 Supplement response ⎫ In cooperation with medically
5 Interrupt response  ⎬ initiated action except in emergency
                       ⎭ or if concerned with monitoring

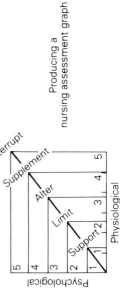

Producing a nursing assessment graph

Responses can be either physiological or psychological.
The graph allows assessment in both areas to identify
priorities of nursing care

Specific nursing actions are determined using nursing skills, knowledge and experience.

You are probably more familiar with one model than others. In that case, go ahead and use that one. We have shown you here that there is more than one model. Do remember to look up the model so that you understand the theory and all the concepts before you try to use that model for a care study.

Each of these models takes a different but related view of illness. Illness is seen as inability to carry out normal activities, inability to self-care or failure to adapt to the stresses of living.

Nursing care is seen as:

1 Assisting with activities of living (Roper)
2 Making up the self-care deficit (Orem)
3 Supporting good adaptation and changing faulty adaptation (Saxton & Hyland).

You will find as a learner that you can use your social skills as a nurse to give effective support to the patient before you have acquired specific theatre skills.

## Care plan

1 You can combine your assessment of the patient with the standard theatre care plan to identify the nursing actions needed for the patient.

2 There may be nursing actions specific to your patient which we have not mentioned so do not forget to include those.

3 Do not forget the specific needs of the operation and the surgeon as these may modify the nursing actions.

4 Deciding the correct nursing action depends on knowledge and experience so you

may need to ask for help from a qualified nurse.

## Evaluation

Points to consider:

1 As the patient is unconscious and very dependent there will be a heavy emphasis on the physical care of the patient. Was this effective? Did this result in any neglect of the psychosocial needs of the patient in the anaesthetic room or the recovery ward – or more particularly, if the patient remained awake during the operation?

2 The interdependence of the theatre team in terms of working together as a team and as the patient moved from one area to another – were good communications maintained?

3 The interdependence of medical and nursing actions to maintain the patient's condition and prevent accidental injury. Differentiate between nursing and medical responsibilities and how they complement each other. Did any of the patient's needs get lost between the two?

4 How important to patient care was good anticipation and preparation in advance?

**Evaluation using a model**
Compare your outcomes and your planned nursing actions.
1 Roper – did the patient maintain his Activities of Living with nursing assistance?
2 Orem – did your nursing actions make up the self-care deficit?
3 Saxton & Hyland – did appropriate nursing action maintain good adaptation responses at each level?

# 14 The role of the theatre nurse

Well, you might have been wondering whether the theatre nurse is a nurse at all. We hope we have shown you that she is. The role of the theatre nurse is to care for the patient before, during and after surgery, to act as a member of a multi-disciplinary team with responsibility for that patient's nursing care whilst he or she is in the operating department. You are to become a member of that team for a short time. Working in a team can show you that it can be fun as well as demanding to work as part of a closely integrated unit. You learn how to discipline your own work to mesh with the other team members in an effective way.

You may miss contact with the patients whilst you are in theatre but do remember that, though we may only see the patient awake for a very short time, it is important that we establish a rapport with him to help him cope with his anxiety at a very stressful time. The support and care that a patient gets in the theatre and recovery area play a vital part in a successful recovery from surgery.

When you finish your experience with us we hope you will have learnt how to help the patient through this very vulnerable period. We also hope that you will have learnt new skills and assimilated new knowledge that will extend your ability to care for the patient before and after surgery.

Quite a number of learners worry that they will not be able to cope with the demands made on them. The theatre staff don't intend to ask too much of anyone but they may occasionally forget that you are still new to the area. If you are asked to do anything which you feel is beyond you, do say so. Never do anything which you have not been taught. Ask for further teaching.

On the other hand, the nature of the work in theatre is such that there are times when it appears that there is nothing going on. If you have some spare time, use it by reading some of the surgical books or journals around the place, investigate the stores to get an idea of where things live, look at and learn the instruments. Instrument catalogues can help you learn. Once again – ask questions of your colleagues.

You will learn a great deal which will be of use to you if you never set foot in a theatre again. A few of you will enjoy your stay so much that you will want to come back when you are qualified.

So, go ahead – enjoy your time in theatre.

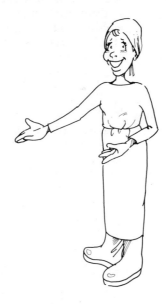

# 15    Theatre procedures

We are very aware that we have hardly mentioned such essential theatre procedures as scrubbing, gowning and gloving, counting swabs, instruments and needles, and safety procedures for using diathermy equipment.

This does not mean that we do not recognise the importance of observing correct procedures to ensure patient safety. Your theatre will almost certainly have written detailed procedures and you will be taught basic theatre techniques before you are allowed to work without supervision.

The National Association of Theatre Nurses produced their 'Codes of Practice' as guidelines for drawing up local theatre procedures. Perhaps there is a copy in your theatre. If there is not and you would like to obtain one, you should write to:

NATN Headquarters
22 Mount Parade
Harrogate

The 'Codes of Practice' cost £1.50.

## FURTHER READING

BINNIE, A. *et al.* 1984. *A Systematic Approach to Nursing Care – An Introduction.* Milton Keynes: Open University Press.

BOORE, J. R. P. 1978. *Prescription for Recovery.* London: Royal College of Nursing.

ELTRINGHAM, R., DURKIN, M. & ANDREWS, S. 1983. *Post-anaesthesia Recovery. A Practical Approach.* Berlin: Springer-Verlag.

GOOCH, J. 1984. *The Other Side of Surgery.* Basingstoke: Macmillan.

HAMILTON SMITH, S. 1972. *Nil by Mouth.* London: Royal College of Nursing.

HAYWARD, J. 1975. *Information – A Prescription against Pain.* London: Royal College of Nursing.

KALIDEEN, D. P. & LEONARD, M. D. 1984. So you're going to have an operation. *NATNEWS,* 22/2 Feb, 12–21.

NATIONAL ASSOCIATION OF THEATRE NURSES. 1982. *Recommended Record of Theatre Experience for Students and Pupil Nurses.* Harrogate: NATN.

NATIONAL ASSOCIATION OF THEATRE NURSES. 1983. *Codes of Practice – Guidelines to Total Patient Care and Safety Practice in Operating Theatres.* Harrogate: NATN.

NIGHTINGALE, K. 1984. Hazards to patients during surgery. No. 1 – pressure injury. *NATNEWS,* 21/9 Sept, 17–18.

OREM, D. 1980. *Nursing: Concepts of Practice.* 2nd Ed. New York: McGraw Hill.

ROPER, N. *et al.* 1985. *The Elements of Nursing.* 2nd Ed. Edinburgh: Churchill Livingstone.

SAXTON, D. & HYLAND, P. A. 1979. *Planning and Implementing Nursing Interventions.* 2nd Ed. St Louis: C. V. Mosby.

WARREN, M. 1981. The total care of a patient within the operating department. *NATNEWS,* 18/4 April, 13–15.

WARREN, M. 1983. *Operating Theatre Nursing.* London: Harper & Row.

# Index

# LEARNING TO CARE SERIES

## General Editors

JEAN HEATH, MED, BA, SRN, SCM, CERT ED
English National Board Learning Resources Unit,
Sheffield

SUSAN E NORMAN, SRN, DNCERT, RNT
Senior Tutor, The Nightingale School, West
Lambeth Health Authority

Titles in this series include:
**Learning to Care for Elderly People**
L THOMAS
**Learning to Care in the Community**
P TURTON and J ORR
**Learning to Care on the ENT Ward**
D STOKES
**Learning to Care in the A&E Department**
G JONES
**Learning to Care in Community Psychiatric Nursing**
M WARD and R BISHOP

**British Library Cataloguing in Publication Data**

Nightingale, Kate
    Learning to care in the theatre. – (Learning to care series)
    1. Operating room nursing
    I. Title
    610.73'677        RD32.3

    ISBN 0 340 39415 3

Typeset in 10/11pt Trump Mediaeval by
Rowland Phototypesetting Ltd, Bury St Edmunds, Suffolk

Printed in Great Britain for Hodder and Stoughton Educational,
a division of Hodder and Stoughton Ltd, Mill Road, Dunton Green,
Sevenoaks, Kent TN13 2YD, by Richard Clay Ltd, Bungay, Suffolk.

# *Learning to care*
## in the
# THEATRE

## Kate Nightingale
### SRN, RMN, RCNT, CertEd,

Nurse Teacher, BUPA Hospital, Norwich
and
The National Association of Theatre Nurses

*with specific contributions by*

Flo Kinnear, RGN, RCNT, RNT DipN (Lond), Nurse Tutor,
St James University Hospital, Leeds

Margaret Heaton, RGN, RCNT, OND, Clinical Nurse Teacher,
Calderdale School of Nursing, Halifax

Doreen Kalideen, SRN, DipN (Lond), RCNT, Clinical Teacher,
ENB Theatre Course 176, Kent and Canterbury Hospital, Canterbury

## HODDER AND STOUGHTON

LONDON   SYDNEY   AUCKLAND   TORONTO